LIVING WITH ALLERGIES

LIVING WITH ALLERGIES

PRACTICAL TIPS FOR ALL THE FAMILY

EMMA AMOSCATO

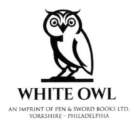

WHITE OWL

AN IMPRINT OF PEN & SWORD BOOKS LTD.
YORKSHIRE – PHILADELPHIA

First published in Great Britain in 2019 by
Pen and Sword White Owl
An imprint of
Pen & Sword Books Ltd
Yorkshire - Philadelphia

Hardback ISBN 978 1 52673 2217
Paperback ISBN 978 1 52675 1607

Typeset in India by Vman Infotech Private Limited

Printed and bound in the UK by TJ International Ltd.

Pen & Sword Books Ltd incorporates the Imprints of Pen & Sword Books Archaeology,
Atlas, Aviation, Battleground, Discovery, Family History, History, Maritime, Military,
Naval, Politics, Railways, Select, Transport, True Crime, Fiction, Frontline Books,
Leo Cooper, Praetorian Press, Seaforth Publishing, Wharncliffe and White Owl.

For a complete list of Pen & Sword titles please contact

PEN & SWORD BOOKS LIMITED
47 Church Street, Barnsley, South Yorkshire, S70 2AS, England
E-mail: enquiries@pen-and-sword.co.uk
Website: www.pen-and-sword.co.uk

or

PEN AND SWORD BOOKS
1950 Lawrence Rd, Havertown, PA 19083, USA
E-mail: Uspen-and-sword@casematepublishers.com
Website: www.penandswordbooks.com

For James and Amalia,
my two allergic adventurers

CONTENTS

FOREWORD

It was a real honour to clinically review this book as it is the first comprehensive book ever on allergy, written by someone who has been on that 'allergic journey' searching for information.

Emma has pulled together so many aspects, covering all the trials and tribulations that people with allergies face and helping to demystify some of the medical jargon.

Knowledge is empowering as it can help us to understand why something happens and what needs to be done about it. It is also important to know that other people live with allergy and to hear their tips and stories, alongside the experts.

This is a really brilliant piece of work for people looking for information on allergy in simple terms and all in one place.

Amena Warner, Clinical Director
Allergy UK

ACKNOWLEDGEMENTS

This book started six years ago when my son, James, turned my world upside down. He made me a mum and unbeknowingly at the time, an allergy mum. Thanks to my NCT friends, who I wouldn't have got through those tough early months without.

The idea grew after I started my blog and connected with other people in the same situation. Thanks to everyone who guided me along the way, to my free from gang for always understanding and particularly to Mel and Rebecca for being my biggest cheerleaders.

Allergy UK have supported the idea of this book from the start and I'm particularly grateful to Amena Warner for her encouragement and enthusiasm and to Dawn Hoy for coordinating my efforts.

I would like to say a huge thanks to all my expert contributors who have not only shared their expertise, but work tirelessly to improve the lives of people with allergies: Rosan Meyers, Dr Neil Shah, Dr Carsten Flohr, Professor Chris Corrigan, Roisin Fitzsimons, Grace Brocklehurst, Dr Stephen Till, Rebecca Knibb, Mary Feeney and Professor George Du Toit.

A special thanks to Dr Adam Fox who has championed the book and who has helped so many other families like us.

This book wouldn't be the same without the invaluable advice from all the people living with allergies: Karen Waggott, Hannah Fouracre, Katharine Spencer, Midge Peacock, Katy Stevens, Suzanne Meadows, Fiona Wood, Chloe Wood, Laura Amoscato, Mel Knibb, Nathalie Newman, Ellie Ludlam, Amy Wobbaka, Rachael Egginton, Lauren Gordon, Clare Hussein, Nina Modak, Chloe Rowland, Callum Newman, Allie Bahn, Kortney Kwong Hing, Hailey Phillips, Freya Spencer, Laura Kenny, Kyle Dine, Emily Chapman, Ruth Holroyd, JP Knibb, Ellie Knibb, Theo Wood and Carly Talbot.

Thanks to my publisher Jonathan for giving me this opportunity, Janet for keeping me on track and Helen Braid for designing me the perfect front cover.

I also want to thank my Allergy Travels team, Allie, Kortney and Kyle who always inspire me and show how my children can grow up and embrace the world with their allergies.

Finally, thanks to my family and my parents for being there every step of the way, James and Amalia for inspiring all that I do and my husband Carl, for always believing in me.

INTRODUCTION

Living with allergies is becoming increasingly common for millions of families across the UK and can be overwhelming, anxiety-inducing and life changing. I know, because we're one of them.

I have two children who between them have multiple allergies, asthma, allergic rhinitis and eczema. It has been a steep learning curve. When they first started showing symptoms and were eventually diagnosed, there were so many things I didn't know and I struggled to find all the information I needed. I scoured the internet, I read studies and factsheets and I reached out to medical professionals. I wanted to know not only how to deal with things now, but also what their future looked like. Would they grow out of them? Could they be cured? How would they cope with school, being a teenager or life as an adult?

I couldn't find a good guide to allergies that covered all the basics in one place and left me feeling informed and inspired. So I decided to write one myself. The subject of allergies is wide and complex and the more I read about it the more I want to discover. It is not possible to cover it all in these pages, but I have tried to give an overview to help you manage your allergies in a practical and proactive way. I have spoken to ten of the country's top allergy experts and hundreds of everyday people living with allergies to bring you the best tips and advice. Allergies don't need to stop you living a fun and full life. They just sometimes mean you need to do things a bit differently.

OUR STORY

When my son was born in 2013, he was an unhappy baby. He cried, he vomited, he slept terribly, developed severe eczema and started losing weight. As a new mum, I was at a loss for what to do. I went to the doctor's multiple times and they kept prescribing emollients and mild steroids to soothe his eczema. They didn't work and no-one was listening. 'Are you a first-time mum?' they would ask in a condescending tone and I was told it was normal for babies to cry and be unsettled.

I was exhausted, upset and desperate to help my baby. I insisted on seeing a new GP who took one look at James and sent us to A&E. The dermatology consultant came down to see us and told me he was going to get the eczema under control. I was so relieved. I asked if his symptoms could be caused by food allergies through my breast milk and he reassured me they couldn't.

I trusted him and carried on breastfeeding with a normal diet. I applied the new steroids and James' skin began to clear up but every time we tried to reduce them, it just flared up again.

Once we started weaning him, it was clear food allergies were the issue and after a severe reaction to hummus, we were finally referred to an allergist. At 9 months old, he tested positive for allergies to milk, egg, peanuts, tree nuts, sesame, garlic, cod, grass pollen and dogs.

We eliminated the foods completely from his diet, his eczema cleared without the need for steroids and soon he was like a different boy. A much happier one.

But it was hard to know what to feed him, how to keep him safe when we were out and how to trust others to care for him. It was an on-the-job learning curve and we started figuring things out along the way.

When he was 14 months old, James took a sip from another child's milk bottle and had an anaphylactic reaction. Within minutes his airways were closing up and he was struggling to breathe. Luckily, we had already been prescribed adrenaline auto-injectors and were able to administer one before calling an ambulance.

It was a terrifying experience and made me even more aware and anxious about keeping him safe. As a journalist, I turned to writing and started a blog FreeFromFarmhouse.com to help document our journey. Soon I found many more people with similar stories and an amazing support network online. I read, I listened and I learnt. I worked out how to cook safe meals, put allergy management plans in places and cope with the psychological impact of allergies.

James also developed asthma and has had multiple hospital trips, nebulisers and steroids. Some of his attacks are viral and others are triggered by pollens or mould, so we have learnt to manage this too.

In 2015, I gave birth to my daughter. I didn't cut any allergens pre-emptively out of my diet to breastfeed her and was determined not to look for symptoms or assume she had allergies too. However, it was obvious immediately that she was following the same path. Still, I had to fight my way to a diagnosis, to a dairy free formula and to an allergy referral.

Amalia had her first severe reaction at 6 months old and has allergies to milk, egg, sesame and chilli. She is also allergic to dogs and cats and has recurrent urticaria.

Happily, we have made some positive progress and James has outgrown his milk allergy after slowly climbing the milk ladder, despite his previous anaphylactic reaction! We have attempted to reintroduce egg a few times with little success but we will continue to take a proactive approach, under guidance from our allergy clinic.

Life with two allergic children can be challenging but it is our normal. We still do everything a regular family would do – we socialise, eat out and travel – but sometimes it just takes a bit more planning and attention to detail to make it happen safely.

Chapter 1

UNDERSTANDING ALLERGIES

What are allergies?

Allergies are the body's immune system responding to a substance (allergen) it sees as a threat. These are usually everyday substances such as food, pollen or animals that do not cause problems for non-allergic people but an allergic person's immune system has become sensitised to them. When the body has an allergic reaction, the immune system goes into overdrive and cells release histamine to attack the threat.

How does your body become sensitised to allergens?

The first time your body comes into contact with an allergen, the immune system decides if it is harmful or not. If it decides it is, then it has become sensitised and antibodies, which usually fight off infection, are ready to attack it the next time you are exposed. The allergen may have entered your body through eating it, breathing it in, through broken skin or your mother's breast milk. This is why children may have an allergic reaction to a food the first time they eat is as the body has recognised it on a previous exposure, which wasn't direct ingestion. Not everyone who becomes sensitised to an allergen will go on to have an allergic reaction though. Studies vary wildly in trying to predict this, concluding anywhere between 11-65 per cent[1] and there is still no real understanding of why some sensitised people develop an allergy and others don't. It is possible to develop an allergy at any time, even after safely consuming or coming into contact with the allergen multiple times before.

A leading hypothesis is that babies are sensitised though their skin at a young age by being exposed to allergens on caregivers' hands or in house dust. Evolutionarily, proteins entering the body through the skin were harmful, e.g. parasites, so the immune system is more likely to gear up to fight them. Babies with bad eczema are statistically more likely to develop allergies. While this may be because they already have atopic tendencies, it is now believed they are more likely to become sensitised to food proteins though their broken skin.

Can babies be born with allergies?

There is a genetic risk and over 30 per cent of children with one allergic or atopic parent and 60-80 per cent of children where both parents have allergic or atopic disease will develop it themselves. You cannot pass on a specific allergy, only the allergic disposition. This compares to just 12 per cent of children with no family history of allergies.[2] There has also been research identifying over 100 genetic risk factors[3]. However, there is no clear evidence whether this genetic disposition can begin from birth, or if the baby needs to be sensitised to the allergen outside the womb first.

What symptoms can allergies cause?

Allergies cause a diverse range of symptoms from minor irritations to life threatening attacks. They mainly affect the respiratory, digestive and circulatory systems, as well as the skin. Symptoms range from eczema, sneezing and watery eyes, to a raised rash called hives, vomiting, breathing difficulties and loss of blood pressure. Most allergies will not cause severe symptoms but can seriously affect people's quality of life, while those at risk of life threatening anaphylactic reactions can face ongoing anxiety.

How common are they?

There has been a rapid rise in allergic disease and it is not slowing down. The percentage of children diagnosed with allergic rhinitis and eczema has trebled over the last 30 years and almost half of the UK population (44%) now suffer from at least one allergy.[4]

Severe reactions are also on the increase and seven times as many people were admitted to hospital with severe allergic reactions in Europe in 2015 than in 2005.[5]

Why are they on the rise?

There are many theories about why allergies are on the rise. Part of it can be explained by the fact there is now more awareness and better diagnosis. Many anaphylactic reactions and deaths used to be categorised as asthmatic or from unknown causes. However, this doesn't account for the dramatic increase, especially in westernised countries.

Allergies are more common in people with an atopic history, where their parents have allergies, asthma or eczema, but why are so many people with no history of allergies facing them?

A popular theory is the hygiene hypothesis. This suggests that our environments are becoming too sterile and devoid of bacteria that our bodies need to develop a strong immune system. When they are not introduced to a range of microbes, they begin to see everyday items as a threat and react irrationally to fight them. This is not just about cleaning too much but also about our food and water being more sanitised, and children not playing outside as much. Children that grow up on farms, or whose pregnant mothers lived on one, are less likely to develop allergies.[6] There is also evidence to show that people with pets are less likely to have allergies – not necessarily because they become desensitised to them, but because the animals introduce different microbes to the home.

Modern living may also be contributing to this as good insulation, central heating and more soft furnishings make an ideal environment for dust mites to flourish.

Our diets also have an influence on developing allergies. The guidance used to be for pregnant women and young children to avoid highly allergenic foods, whereas now it is believed that avoiding them may actually contribute to developing allergies. (see more: chapter 17) Beyond that, the over processing and sterility of our food may all be harming our gut bacteria and making us more susceptible to allergies. Antibiotics in early life, or during pregnancy, and being delivered by caesarean section are also risk factors as these too can weaken the gut bacteria.

Another theory is that a lack of vitamin D during infancy and the mother's pregnancy, from less outdoor activity and sun exposure, is contributing to children developing allergies. Some studies suggest that children born in the autumn or winter are more likely to develop allergies.[7] A study in the *Journal of Allergy and Clinical Immunology* showed babies with low vitamin D were three times more likely to have food allergies.

'With identical twins, sharing the same pregnancy, same time in special baby care, same earlier years environments and same weaning and early years diet - yet only one has allergies - it is clear to me that there is no easy answer to the question of what causes allergies.'
Karen Waggott

Can allergies be cured?

There is currently no cure for allergies, although immunotherapies can help reduce the severity and likelihood of reactions as they desensitise the immune system. (see more: chapter 8) Allergies are generally managed by limiting or avoiding contact with the substance causing the allergic reaction and preventing or treating any symptoms they cause.

Can you outgrow them?

It is possible to outgrow allergies at any age, although it is most common in childhood. Most young children (up to 80%) with milk and egg allergies outgrow these by age five. The less severe the symptoms, the earlier the first reaction and the less prevalence of eczema, the higher chance there is of outgrowing it. There is much less chance of outgrowing other allergies such as peanuts and tree nuts, with the rate being closer to 20 per cent. Once a child enters adolescence, it is more likely that their allergies will be lifelong.

How likely are you to develop others?

Overall, nearly half of people with one allergic condition will also have another.[8] For those who have food allergies, around 30 per cent will develop another one[9] Risk factors include family history and early onset eczema. It is possible for people to develop allergies at any age and is more common after illness or hormonal changes. It is also possible to redevelop allergies you have grown out of or reduce tolerance after reducing exposure – for example, being away from the family pet at university. Children with a food allergy are also more than twice as likely to have asthma and more than three times as likely to have respiratory allergy or eczema.

How likely are you to have a further child with allergies?

There is no predicting whether a subsequent child will have allergies. You are more likely to have a child with allergies if one or both parents have them; however, having one child with allergies does not increase the risk of a sibling developing them.

'Second time around it was easier – easier to spot the symptoms, easier to get help. My two children's allergies aren't all the same, the symptoms aren't the same and the levels of severity for different allergens aren't the same. But our ability to cope, to know which foods aren't safe, the questions to ask when eating out, how to talk to childcare providers about care plans – it was all easier second time around. You have protected one child and you have enough confidence and "know how" how to cope the next time. As siblings, they too will be able to look out for each other and help keep each other stay safe as they grow.'
Hannah Fouracre

Chapter 2

FOOD ALLERGIES

Food allergies occur when the body mistakenly identifies proteins in food as a threat and triggers its defence system. It is estimated that 5-8 per cent children have a food allergy and 1-2 per cent adults.[1] It is possible to be allergic to any food but the most common are milk, soy and egg in infancy, and peanuts, tree nuts and shellfish in later life.

IgE-mediated food allergies

In IgE-mediated food allergies, the immune system becomes sensitised to a food protein and sees it as a threat. It then produces immunoglobulin E antibodies (IgE) to fight it. These antibodies release chemicals, including histamine, from mast cells in the body to fight the threat and cause a range of symptoms. These can include hives (a raised rash), itchiness, swelling, vomiting and breathing difficulties. These reactions usually happen immediately or within a couple of hours of eating the food and in extreme cases, can cause a severe, life-threatening reaction called anaphylaxis when histamine is released into the bloodstream. (see more: chapter 7)

People with IgE-mediated food allergies usually need to avoid that food completely. They also need to be aware of the risks of cross-contamination in cooking and food preparation as in some cases, trace amounts can cause a severe reaction.

'Try and remember that things will get easier. At first diagnosis, there is so much information to take in and being overwhelmed is completely normal. However, as you go through your allergy journey, it does get easier to deal with. Focus on what your child can eat not what they can't eat. This was the best piece of advice I was given. It really turned a scary, lonely and unknown situation into a more positive light.'
Katharine Spencer

Non IgE-mediated food allergies

Non IgE-mediated allergies are also caused by the immune system but do not involve antibodies. Non IgE allergies cause inflammation in the body and symptoms tend to be delayed and begin after a few hours and up to 72 hours later. They can include reflux, colic, vomiting, eczema, abdominal pain, diarrhoea or blood in the stools. Symptoms take longer to resolve than IgE reactions as the body can react until the system has cleared the food protein. Non-IgE reactions do not cause anaphylaxis.

Many people will need to avoid these foods completely, while others may be able to tolerate small amounts without a reaction.

Many people will only have IgE or non-IgE reactions, but it is possible to have a mix of both to different foods and concentrations of the allergen.

'The hardest thing about managing Non-IgE allergies is getting people around you to understand that they need to be taken seriously. Particularly if it is your children that suffer from them. People just see the lack of a reaction immediately or an auto-injector and assume that it doesn't need to be catered for. What they don't see is the knock on effect and just how drained you feel afterwards. After a delayed reaction we top up with multi-vitamins, drink plenty of water and are careful about seeing people with germs as we find that we are more susceptible to them.'
Midge Peacock

Oral allergy syndrome (OAS)

Oral Allergy Syndrome is an allergy to certain pollens that cross react with raw fruits or vegetables that have similar proteins. This usually results in an itchy and uncomfortable mouth or mild swelling of the tongue or throat and reactions are often worse during the pollen season. Cooking these fruits and vegetables changes the proteins and most people can then tolerate them. People with OAS can also react in the same way to nuts, so it is important to rule out whether a reaction is an IgE-mediated allergy. OAS is very rarely anaphylactic and symptoms usually subside within 30 minutes by drinking water or taking an antihistamine. The most common pollen in the UK is birch pollen which cross reacts with a lot of foods. (see: table 1)

Food Protein-Induced Gastroenteritis Syndrome (FPIES)

Food Protein-Induced Gastroenteritis Syndrome (FPIES) affects the gastrointestinal tract and symptoms, which usually present 2-3 hours after ingestion, can include severe vomiting, diarrhoea and dehydration. This can lead to extreme lethargy, a drop in blood pressure and shock. There is often a delay in diagnosis as symptoms can mimic an infection and causes cannot be picked up through allergy testing, only elimination. The most common triggers are cow's milk and soy, followed by rice and oats, but any food protein can be a cause.

FPIES reactions can be severe and it is important to get fluids quickly. This condition is often misunderstood by medical professionals and it can be a good idea to prepare a letter to take to A&E explaining the condition. FPIES usually resolves with time.

'My GP dismissed my fears about my daughter. At 10 days old he told me "all babies are sick". At 5 months old he told me she "didn't look ill". Getting diagnosed was a process of elimination for us and by 16 months it was evident that it was FPIES purely from Daisy's reactions and hospital admissions.'   *Katy Stevens*

Eosinophilic Gastrointestinal Disorders (EOS/EGID)

Eosinophilic Gastrointestinal Disorders (EGID) are caused by increased amounts of eosinophils, a type of white blood cell, in the gastrointestinal tract. They are a response to a food allergy and can cause inflammation and tissue damage. Eosinophilic Oesophagitis (EOE) is the most common disorder and occurs in the oesophagus (food pipe). It can cause problems swallowing, vomiting, reflux and failure to thrive. EGIDs are diagnosed by an endoscopy where a camera is inserted in the gastrointestinal tract and small biopsies are taken to check for eosinophils.

EGIDs are treated by eliminating the allergenic foods. If this is proving difficult, you may be advised to move onto an elemental formula to help the body recover. Corticosteroids and some anti-reflux medication may also help.

Food intolerances

There is still a lot of confusion about the difference between allergies and intolerances, especially with non-IgE allergies. Food intolerances do not involve the immune system and tend to cause symptoms such as bloating, change in bowel movements, IBS, lethargy or skin problems. Some people may be able to tolerate small amounts of a food but have adverse reactions when they consume more. The incidence of food allergies is often over-reported. A study on the Isle of Wight showed 34 per cent reported food allergies in their children but only 5 per cent actually had a true allergy.[2]

Lactose intolerance

Lactose intolerance is not the same as a milk allergy and occurs when the gut doesn't produce the right enzymes to break down the lactose (milk sugars). Symptoms often include bloating, stomach cramps and diarrhoea. It is very rare that a baby is lactose intolerant as it usually takes a number of years for the enzymes to stop working. Lactose intolerance is usually diagnosed by an elimination diet but your doctor may also suggest a hydrogen breath test or glucose blood test.

Histamine intolerance

Histamine is a chemical which your immune system releases to attack an allergen. However, it is possible to have too much in your body and this can cause adverse symptoms including headaches, nausea, hives, angioedema (swelling) and fatigue. Some symptoms of histamine intolerance mimic a true allergic reaction but it is not IgE-mediated. It is usually caused by a build-up of histamine in the foods you are eating, rather than your body over-releasing it.

There is no reliable test for histamine intolerance and it is usually diagnosed after investigating other possible causes and keeping a food diary to identify symptom patterns.

If you suffer from histamine intolerance then you will need to limit your intake of high histamine foods including: alcohol, dried food, tinned or pickled foods, cured meats, and some legumes and vegetables. Some other foods also act as histamine releasers and will also need to be avoided.

Coeliac disease

Coeliac disease is not an allergy but an autoimmune condition where the immune system reacts to gluten. This causes damage to the lining of the gut which makes it difficult to absorb nutrients and can lead to further complications. It is important to be tested for coeliac disease if you have unexplained weight loss, ongoing fatigue, mouth ulcers, anaemia or unexplained stomach issues and if positive, avoid gluten completely.

Expert Insight: Non-IgE Allergies

Neil Shah
Paediatric Gastroenterologist
Great Ormond Street Hospital

How can people recognise non-IgE allergies?

The majority of non-IgE allergies are caused by dairy, soya, egg and wheat. It's difficult to recognise symptoms as many common ones may not be related to food. A combination of reflux, colic, a change in bowel movement, blood in the stools, vomiting and stomach pain can all indicate an allergy but one on its own is unlikely to be. Risk factors for non-IgE allergies include family history, eczema, being born by caesarean and the use of antibiotics in early life.

Parents often face difficulties getting a diagnosis – why is this?

We are still working through the best ways to look for, test and treat non-IgE. We're seeing a big increase in allergies in general, but some people can be very dismissive of delayed allergies. They can have a huge impact on quality of life – a lack of sleep and watching your child in constant pain or not eating is extremely difficult. There are often very few external signs and GPs dismiss the idea of an allergy if the child is not losing weight but actually this is a very poor marker. It is quite uncommon to lose weight with a milk allergy. Good evidence-based guidelines are lacking and recognition and training needs to improve at primary care level upwards.

When can parents start reintroducing foods?

Parents can be nervous about attempting reintroductions and see it as poisoning or harming their child, but it is important not to restrict the diet any more than necessary. Reintroductions should only be trialled when a child is well. Most people can start trialling milk from the age of one and most will resolve by the age of three but not everyone recovers. It's going to get better though. People can lose sight of that. The toughest time is when they are youngest.

Are people with non-IgE allergies more likely to develop other conditions?

Milk allergy interfaces with other atopic conditions like asthma and eczema. The probability of allergies leading to other gut problems and IBS is higher if they are left untreated.

Do probiotics play a role in treating or preventing non-IgE allergies?

Gut bacteria is key to lots of diseases and the role of probiotics is going to be key for lots of conditions including allergies. Newer pathways are looking at stabilising, repairing and healing the gut. Key long-term issues also include maternal probiotics, how children are delivered and the use of antibiotics. We also need to be careful not to over-restrict the diet and reintroduce foods as soon as possible.

Why do some people develop allergies later in life?

Many people develop allergies to food post-infection or after things like gastroenteritis. Whatever destabilises the gut. Research and understanding into non-IgE allergies is still way behind but these are exciting times and we will get there. The understanding of the overlap with IBS is also improving and this makes for an interesting future in the management of children and adults with food reactive gut symptoms.

Chapter 3

ENVIRONMENTAL AND OTHER ALLERGIES

Many allergens are not directly ingested but enter the body through the airways or skin. These are often referred to as environmental allergens or aeroallergens. They can be more difficult to manage as it is almost impossible to avoid them completely and usually cause chronic symptoms including skin irritation or allergic rhinitis, as well as triggering asthma and eczema.

Animals

It is possible to be allergic to any animal, although cats and dogs are often the most troublesome as they are most likely to be kept as pets. Animal allergies most commonly cause itchy eyes, sneezing or skin irritation as well as respiratory symptoms. The allergens can be found in the animal's saliva and in their dander, which is the skin cells they have shed. You may be allergic to one or both of these. Some breeds of animals produce less dander than others and are less likely to cause allergic reactions, but it is not possible to have a truly allergen-free or hypoallergenic cat or dog.

House dust mites

House dust mites are one of the most common causes of allergies and trigger eczema, asthma and allergic rhinitis. They have been shown to cause reactions in up to 85 per cent of children with asthma.[1] They are the miniscule creatures which live in the dust in our home and feed mainly off shed skin cells. It is their droppings that are inhaled and cause symptoms. It is very difficult to remove dust mites completely, especially in warm and humid conditions in UK houses, as they usually linger in carpets, upholstery and bedding.

Moulds

Moulds can be found in outdoor and indoor environments and flourish in damp, warm conditions like bathrooms and kitchens. They produce spores which are very fine and airborne so are easy to breathe in and are released when the temperature in a damp environment rapidly increases. Symptoms, which are usually respiratory, can come on quickly especially if the spores trigger asthma, or produce a more chronic response of sneezing, watery eyes or itching if you are regularly exposed to them.

Pollen

Pollen is high in protein and very fine which means it is very allergenic and difficult to completely avoid. It creates a lot of discomfort and upset for many people and as well as causing allergic rhinitis (hay fever) can also trigger asthma attacks and eczema flare ups. There are many different pollens which flower at varying time throughout the year, so it is important to try and understand which affect you. 95 per cent of people suffering from hay fever will find grass pollen (May to July) is a trigger, while tree pollen (February to June) and weed (June to September) can also affect people.

Other allergies

Food and environmental allergens are not the only things that can trigger an allergic reaction. Other common substances can cause anaphylaxis or ongoing distress.

Drugs

Lot of drugs have side effects such as itching or nausea and it can be difficult to know if your symptoms are one of them, or a true allergy. Some drugs such as penicillin and some anaesthetics are known to be more likely to cause allergic reactions and NSAIDs such as asprin or ibuprofen are the next most likely. Up to 1 in 10 people claim to have a penicillin allergy but only around 10% of those actually do.[3] This is often due to them being labelled allergic after a skin rash or mild symptoms while taking the drug in childhood. Drug reactions can be mild and just cause urticaria or itchiness but are also one of the leading causes of anaphylaxis. If you are unsure, stop taking the drug immediately and contact your GP who may refer you for further testing. You may be able to take other drugs in the same group or need to avoid them completely.

If you know you are allergic to a drug, then make sure it is clearly flagged in your medical records. Tell anyone who is treating you and make sure you are given an allergy bracelet in hospital.

Latex

People can react to the proteins in latex which can cause two distinct types of reaction. One is a delayed skin reaction, contact dermatitis, which causes an itchy red rash. The other is an immediate IgE-mediated response which can lead to anaphylaxis.

Balloons, condoms and latex gloves can all cause problems and latex can also be found in everyday items like erasers, sports equipment and hot water bottles. Latex gloves coated with powder can also cause airborne reactions but are now banned in most hospital settings and this alone has led to a decrease in severe reactions. Some foods, including bananas, avocado and kiwi fruit share similar proteins to latex, so people may be likely to cross-react.

'Everyday places can be a huge risk with a latex allergy; the dentist, doctors, hospital all pose a risk with the use of latex gloves and I have to remember to check with them before any treatment. In bakers, butchers etc again I have to be careful that latex gloves do not touch my food. As a grown woman I still have to be very careful and aware when taking my children to parties because of balloons, even if I go out on a night out there's usually someone out with balloons.'   *Suzanne Meadows*

Insect stings

The venom released in insect stings can cause localised reactions or lead to swelling and itchiness beyond the initial sting site and throughout the limb. These symptoms can usually be treated with antihistamines and oral steroids. Children experiencing non-localised reactions are unlikely to be at risk of more severe ones, but this kind of response usually indicates a higher risk in adults. Insect stings can, in rare cases, cause anaphylaxis which is more common in people who have regular contact with wasps or bees in their work.

Nickel

Nickel allergy usually presents as eczema or dermatitis after prolonged contact with the skin, so most often when wearing jewellery. Platinum, 18ct gold or solid silver are usually fine but lower grade metal can cause problems. Brief contact with other metals, like kitchen implements, rarely cause any irritation. Some people may develop an allergy to foods containing a high amount of nickel such as broccoli, chocolate, tea and canned food and will need to avoid these as well.

Chemicals and fragrances

People can be allergic to many different chemicals but a reasonably common one is paraphenylenediamine, which is found in hair dyes. This is most likely to cause localised irritation or swelling but can also lead to anaphylaxis. Other chemicals in hair dyes, as well as in black henna tattoos, can also cause reactions.

It is also possible to have multiple chemical sensitivity and react to fragrances, including perfumes. The most common symptoms are difficulty breathing, itchy eyes and throat, or congestion and headaches. People need to find fragrance free or natural alternatives to cleaning, bathing and cosmetic products. It can be almost impossible to avoid fragrances and chemicals outside the home and can be very challenging, so symptoms are usually managed with daily medication.

'I was told my symptoms were from an allergy to perfumes and fragrances so out went the shampoo, conditioner, body wash, deodorants, soap, washing up liquid, cleaning products, room plugin, air freshener, candles, oil burner etc. At that point, I could not believe how much our world was full of scents and smells.'   *Fiona Wood*

Occupational allergies

Occupational allergies develop when someone is exposed to ongoing amounts of a substance through their workplace. They may not have had any reactions to this substance before, but their body becomes sensitised through ongoing exposure.

Industries which are commonly at risk for occupational allergies include:

- Food processing
- Vehicle spray painting
- Working with animals
- Healthcare
- Baking
- Woodworking

- Hairdressing
- Floristry
- Beekeeping

People can develop a range of symptoms from allergic asthma, rhinitis and contact dermatitis, to anaphylactic reactions. Immunotherapy is available to treat some occupational allergies, but others will need to be managed with medication or in extreme cases, a change of career.

Chapter 4

ECZEMA AND SKIN ALLERGIES

Atopic eczema

Atopic eczema, or atopic dermatitis, is fairly common, especially in children. It is caused by an impaired skin barrier that leads to dry, itchy skin and inflammation. Symptoms can vary greatly in severity from mild dry and flaky patches in limited areas to red, irritated, infected skin that is widespread across the body.

Atopic eczema has a genetic link and it usually begins in the first year of life. Many children will grow out of it or their symptoms will lessen, although it can persist into adulthood. Eczema cannot be cured but it can be managed relatively effectively in most cases by avoiding any triggers and having a good treatment plan.

Eczema and food allergies

Children that have moderate to severe eczema in their first few months of life are more likely to develop a food allergy. This may partly be because they have a higher genetic disposition to it, but recent studies also suggest that the broken skin allows food proteins to enter the bloodstream. This causes the immune system to recognise them as harmful and become sensitised, which may then lead to an allergic response when the food is later ingested.

Food allergies cannot cause eczema, but they can be a strong trigger, especially in young children. A food can trigger an eczema flare up within minutes of eating or as a delayed reaction. The most common food triggers are dairy and wheat. Sometimes, addressing these food allergies and cutting them out can clear up the eczema completely without the need for further treatment.

Other eczema triggers

As well as foods, there are many other common allergens that can trigger eczema flares. Environmental allergens such as dust mites, pollens and animal dander can all make it worse while chemicals in cosmetics and cleaning products can also be a problem. Many people's eczema is also sensitive to heat, cold or changes in temperature and can be made worse by exposure to water which dries the skin.

Contact dermatitis

Contact dermatitis is where eczema is triggered by the skin touching an allergen or irritant. Common triggers are nickel (found in lots of jewellery), cosmetic ingredients, plants or topical medicines.

If you suspect an allergy is triggering eczema or contact dermatitis, then you should be referred to a specialist for testing.

'Managing eczema and environmental allergies is tough but once you find a regime that fits your lifestyle it all becomes so much easier. I have regular medication alarms on my phone so that I never forget to administer antihistamine and we always check pollen levels before a big day out. Indoor allergens such as dust are out worst enemy, but I hoover once or twice a day with our HEPA filter hoover before damp dusting all surfaces. It may seem very daunting but once you find your rhythm you'll wonder what you were so worried about.' *Chloe Wood*

Urticaria

Urticaria is the medical term for nettle rash or hives, a raised and usually itchy rash that can appear across the body. Acute urticaria, that comes on suddenly, is an IgE mediated reaction and is caused by having contact with or ingesting an allergen. It usually resolves on its own or with antihistamine within an hour but can develop into more severe, life threatening symptoms.

Chronic or recurrent urticaria is not usually caused by allergies. Sometimes it is viral or an overreaction of the body's immune system. Other people will experience physical urticaria which is a response to extremes of temperature or pressure. It is also possible to have aquagenic or solar urticaria, where your skin reacts to water or the sun in a similar way with a widespread itchy rash. This kind of urticaria can be very uncomfortable but will usually calm down once the skin stops being exposed. It is rarely IgE mediated and therefore unlikely to develop further into anaphylaxis.

Angioedema

Angioedema is the swelling of the body, lips, face, or tongue. Acute angioedema is a symptom of an allergic reaction and may present with urticaria, alone or with other symptoms, as part of an anaphylactic reaction. Chronic angioedema, like urticaria, is not usually allergy-induced and often has no clear trigger. Chronic urticaria and angioedema can cause a lot of discomfort and upset and also exacerbate other skin conditions such as eczema.

These chronic conditions are usually managed by avoiding any triggers and taking antihistamines or steroids to reduce the symptoms.

Contact reactions

It is possible to have acute contact reactions to food or other allergens when they touch the skin, even if the allergen is not ingested. Usually this will just cause hives or localised swelling but in rare cases it can progress to anaphylaxis. In younger children, this may be more likely if they transfer the allergen to their eyes or mouth through contact. Some high histamine or acidic food, like tomatoes, can cause similar skin reactions but are not indicative of an allergy.

Expert Insight: Eczema and allergies

Dr Carsten Flohr
Head, Unit for Population-Based Dermatology Research, St John's Institute of Dermatology,
Guy's & St Thomas' NHS Foundation Trust

What is the link between eczema and allergies?

Current thinking is that eczema is the 'gateway' to food allergies and in some ways, respiratory allergies. The skin is the first line of defence and in early life, food proteins can make contact with the immune system through the broken and inflamed skin in eczema and sensitise the immune system, leading to food allergies. While there is good scientific evidence for this from research in animals and humans for food allergies, further studies are needed to provide evidence for airborne allergies, such as to house dust mite, grass and tree pollen.

What can parents do to prevent this?

There appears to be a very important window of opportunity to stop eczema and prevent allergies by preventing skin barrier breakdown in early life. One easy approach is for parents to use emollients on their babies from birth. Also, data from the EAT (Enquiring About Tolerance) study shows children living in a hard water area (higher domestic water calcium carbonate concentration) have a significantly higher risk of developing eczema compared to those living in soft water areas. There may therefore be benefit installing water softeners in high risk families before a child is born and this is currently being tested in the Softened Water for Eczema Prevention (SOFTER) trial led by the Paediatric Dermatology Department at Guy's & St Thomas' Hospital.

Can food allergies trigger eczema?

Yes, especially in early life food allergies can be an important flare factor for eczema, especially where the eczema starts during the first 6 months of life and does not adequately respond to optimal skin care and topical treatments.

What role do environmental allergies play?

Environmental triggers are often difficult to identify. House dust mite sensitisation is common in children with significant eczema but impossible to eradicate completely. Dogs and cats are less common triggers, and there is evidence that owning a dog during the first year of life provides a degree of protection against eczema development. The opposite seems true for cats.

How likely are children to outgrow eczema?

About 60 per cent of children outgrow their eczema by adolescence but this is less likely if they have early onset, more severe eczema as well as food allergies and/or respiratory allergies. The atopic march which was always thought of as a clear pathway from eczema to food allergies and then respiratory allergies has turned out to be a bit of myth. Only around 10 per cent children follow this classical pattern while there are many more permutations.

Is there a link between gut health and eczema?

There is good evidence that children with reduced microbiome diversity in early life have a higher likelihood of developing eczema. The link between the skin and the gut immune systems is less well understood but the research suggests that giving probiotics in the third trimester and in early life reduces the risk of eczema development by around 50 per cent. We are currently studying the link between the microbiome of the gut and the skin as well as eczema and food allergies in the EAT Study.

Chapter 5

RESPIRATORY ALLERGIES

Respiratory allergies are when the body has an allergic response to a substance that is breathed in, also known as an aeroallergen. These can cause a range of symptoms from itchy eyes, sneezing and congestion to worsening asthma, but rarely cause anaphylaxis.

Aeroallergens can include pollens, moulds, house dust mites and animals. Whereas pollens tend to be seasonal, indoor allergens like dust mites can persist year round.

Asthma

Asthma is a condition where the airways are sensitive and when something irritates them they are more likely to become tight or inflamed, making it difficult to breathe. Asthma is more common in atopic families and affects 5.4 million people in the UK: 1 in 11 children and 1 in 12 adults.[1] Eczema and food allergies, especially egg allergy in infancy, are both risk factors for developing asthma.

Symptoms include:

- Wheezing
- Persistent cough
- Chest tightness
- Shortness of breath

Most asthma symptoms build up over a period of time but during an asthma attack may worsen quickly. You or your child may find breathing difficult, be unable to finish a sentence without taking a breath or in younger children you may notice their stomach muscles or intercostal muscles (between their ribs) going in and out excessively.

Most asthma is triggered by a virus, temperature change or exercise, but people can also suffer from allergic asthma. Up to 10 per cent of children who suffer asthma attacks may have an allergic trigger, according to Allergy

UK. Common allergic triggers include house dust mites, animals, pollen and moulds. Other irritants such as smoke, weather changes or pollution can also make asthma worse.

It is important that asthma is well managed and regularly reviewed as uncontrolled asthma can make an allergic reaction more severe and is a risk factor for severe or fatal reactions.

'Managing allergic asthma is hard as it is easy to get complacent. Don't let it dictate your life but be realistic. It's about knowing your limits and finding balance. For me that means switching long walks in the countryside in the winter for the short strolls by the sea in the summer when the pollen is high.'   *Midge Peacock*

Viral wheeze

It is rare for doctors to diagnose asthma in children under five. This is because many children suffer from coughs or wheezes when they get a virus as their respiratory system is still developing and their airways are narrow. It is more likely your child will go on to develop asthma if there is a family history, they cough a lot at night, have other symptoms such as breathlessness or if it seems to be triggered by an allergy.

Airborne food allergies

It is possible for people with food allergies to react to small particles of food which have become airborne. This may be when milk is frothed in a cafe, people crack open seafood and the juices spray out, or if someone opens a bag of nuts and the dust escapes. It is rare to have an anaphylactic reaction to airborne food particles and is more likely to happen when a large amount is released from multiple sources in an enclosed environment.

These reactions cannot happen from simply smelling a food as the proteins are not in the scent and most people can safely be around other people eating their allergens. A small scale study found that children with severe peanut allergies could sniff peanut butter without any respiratory or anaphylactic reactions.[2]

Allergic rhinitis

Allergic rhinitis is when IgE antibodies trigger the release of histamine in the nose in response to an aeroallergen such as pollen or pet dander. Symptoms include sneezing, itchy and watery eyes, nasal congestion, tiredness and headaches. It can also cause a cough or wheeze – particularly in patients who also have asthma. It is a problem for up to 30 per cent of adults and 40 per cent of children and can have adverse effects on sleep, quality of life and school performance. Allergic rhinitis is also a major risk factor for developing asthma and around 80 per cent of asthmatics suffer from it, making the condition more difficult to control.[3]

Allergic rhinitis that happens seasonally in response to pollens is more commonly known as hay fever.

> 'My advice is, see a specialist and see them early. Then keep seeing them. I wish I had done that sooner. I spent a long time being sick and feeling bad when I don't think I had to. There are people who specialise in allergies and asthma. Go and see them. Let them teach you things. I learned I'd been using my inhaler wrong my entire life. I watch pharmacists show people how to use inhalers incorrectly. It's so frustrating. There are things that can help. I have a rescue inhaler and now I know when and how to use it. I take a daily drug that helps my breathing. I have immunotherapy that allows me to do things I couldn't do before. I can be outside when things are blooming and I'm not miserable.' *Laura Amoscato*

Expert Insight: Asthma, allergies and allergic rhinitis

Chris Corrigan
Professor of Asthma, Allergy & Respiratory Science
King's College London

What is the relationship between asthmas and allergies?

When I started in the 80s, asthma was seen as an allergic disease. In the 30 years I've been researching it though, I've come to believe it is primarily a disease caused by twitchiness of the smooth muscle which forms the outside lining of the airways and inflammation and swelling of the inner lining of the airways, both of which cause narrowing. The inflammation can be set off by a number of things present in the inhaled air: viruses; pollutants; smoke, etc. Over 80 per cent of asthma is virally triggered. Respiratory viral infections increase the inflammation, twitchiness and blockage of the airways. Allergens such as pollens inhaled in the air can play a role in some asthmatics and stimulate twitchy airways to constrict, which they wouldn't in non-asthmatics.

How does an asthma attack differ from an anaphylactic reaction involving the airways?

Acute asthma usually builds up and people are progressively wheezier or shorter of breath over hours or days as the inflammation in their airways increases. An anaphylactic reaction is a sudden, global histamine release usually triggered by exposure to allergen that can lead to broncho-constriction in existing asthmatics, but rarely in non-asthmatics. An anaphylactic reaction is usually associated with other signs and symptoms at the same time.

How does allergic rhinitis fit into the allergy spectrum?

Allergic rhinitis – or seasonal hay fever – is when the body reacts to inhaled aeroallergens and the mast cells in the nose and eyes release histamine. It is a separate disease but there is an increased incidence of it in people with asthma, eczema or other allergic problems. It can have a big effect on people's quality of life. People can wake up with eyes so swollen they can hardly see and it has been proven to reduce school performance. In some people with hay fever and asthma, their asthma may be worse when their hay fever is bad because of inflammation further down the airways.

How can people best manage their symptoms?

We spend a lot of time explaining and showing people how to do this as it makes a big difference. Many asthma attacks unfortunately happen because people still do not take their inhalers regularly or know how to use them properly. This is essential. For hay fever, people must take antihistamines and steroid nose sprays every day during the pollen season (or all the time if they are troubled by allergens present all the year round) for them to be fully effective. People with asthma also need to be confident to know what to do when things go astray and have a clear plan of action worked out with their carers.

When can people access immunotherapies?

For some people, who still have significant unbearable symptoms to tree or grass pollens, or dust mites even after taking standard medicines (antihistamines and steroid nose sprays) regularly and correctly we can offer immunotherapy. This is given by injection into the arm (typically about 6 injections given every week in the winter for 3 years for pollens and every 6 weeks or so for dust mite) or under the tongue as drops or tablets (must be taken typically every day for 3 years). This raises the threshold of sensitivity to the allergen, making symptoms typically 50-70 per cent better. It is not a cure and does not allow most people to stop taking standard medicines. We also offer it for animal allergies too if people need it for their work – not so they can just keep their pets!

Chapter 6

DIAGNOSIS

The process of diagnosing and treating allergies can be frustrating. This is partly because there can be a lack of understanding in primary care and also because allergy services across the country are stretched and it can be difficult to get a timely referral to a specialist. Some allergies can be easier to diagnose than others. Tests can work well to confirm IgE-mediated reactions but are not always reliable in diagnosing them when used alone and cannot predict the severity of a reaction, while non-IgE-mediated food allergies can only be diagnosed through an elimination diet.

Other allergic conditions, such as FPIES, are often misunderstood or more common conditions like allergic rhinitis, not taken seriously.

There are lots of allergy or intolerance tests available to buy online or from different practitioners including hair or stool analysis, vega testing and kinesiology. None of these have been scientifically proven and cannot test for true food allergies. They may show suspected intolerances, but the results can highlight a long list of foods and encourage you to restrict your diet unnecessarily. Allergy testing should only be done through a licensed medical practitioner.

If you are concerned that you are allergic to something, then it is important to avoid it and contact your GP.

Past reactions

The first thing your doctor will ask you about is any past reactions you have had, what your symptoms were and if there were any obvious triggers. If you have photos, or written records of reactions then take these along with you. If you believe your reaction was triggered by a food, drug or other item such as cosmetics, then take along a list of ingredients to check.

Medical history

You will probably also be asked about your medical history, such as eczema or asthma symptoms as well as whether there are any allergic or atopic diseases in your family. This does not predict or rule out the likelihood of an allergy, but it will help your doctor understand more about your reactions.

Food diaries and elimination

For suspected non-IgE food allergies, your doctor may ask you to keep a food diary if it is difficult to pinpoint what is causing your symptoms or if you seem to be having delayed reactions. This will involve keeping a detailed record of everything you or your child eat and any symptoms you have, along with specific timings. This may help identify a pattern, but it can be hampered by illness, teething or other factors so may not be totally clear.

The next step is to remove any suspected allergens from your diet for at least 2-4 weeks to see if symptoms improve. To confirm a non-IgE allergy, it may be necessary to trial reintroductions after this but you should seek the support of a doctor or dietician to do this. (see more: chapter 16)

Referrals

Many allergies can be dealt with by your GP, who can prescribe medications and help you manage any symptoms. However, it may be necessary to get a referral to a specialist allergy service if your symptoms are causing persistent problems, are uncontrolled by the medications your GP can prescribe, or you may be at risk of anaphylaxis

If your doctor believes you have suffered an IgE-mediated reaction causing an immediate reaction to food, drugs or another substance, then they should refer you for additional testing. The National Institute for Health And Care Excellence (NICE) have clear guidelines on when and how this should happen. (see: resources). If you are not getting the support you think you need, then it is a good idea to take a copy of these along to your GP to strengthen your request.

If they suspect a non-IgE-mediated food allergy, then they will be likely to suggest an elimination diet but should refer you to a dietician for support. If non-IgE reactions are more complicated, have multiple facets or are causing severe symptoms, like failure to thrive in young children, then a referral should be made to a specialist.

Waiting times can be long and there are regional difficulties in accessing allergy clinics as provision varies greatly across the country. So some people may choose to pay for a private appointment. Make sure your allergist is certified by the British Society of Allergy and Clinical Immunology (BSACI) – you can search for an allergy clinic regionally or by condition on their website.

Allergy clinic

When you arrive at the allergy clinic you or your child will be weighed and measured. You will then see one of the allergy team. They will ask you some questions about your medical history, previous reactions and what has led you there, so they can get a better understanding of your allergies. After that, it is likely they will send you for further tests. They will probably do these on the day, especially if they are carrying out skin prick tests which have immediate results, or may make another appointment.

The results of these tests will help them decide what to do next. You will be given an action plan outlining which allergens to avoid and what to do if a reaction takes place. If you are at risk of anaphylaxis, they will prescribe adrenaline auto-injectors and should show you how to use them properly. If results are inconclusive, they may suggest you undertake a challenge or reintroduction.

Allergy tests

Allergy tests should not be confused with intolerance tests. Allergy tests are only available through trained medical professionals who can accurately interpret the results. They will only show up IgE-mediated allergies and are unable to diagnose non-IgE reactions.

Allergy tests can be used for allergies to food, pollen, drugs, moulds and many other substances.

Skin prick tests (SPTs)

Skin prick tests are a quick and straightforward way to see if someone is sensitised to a substance by detecting the level of IgE antibodies in the skin. The allergist will have a range of common allergens that have been extracted into a liquid format. Sometimes, if your allergen is less common, is to a fruit or vegetable, or they want to test it in a certain form, they may ask you to bring a fresh sample from home.

The allergist will then label your arm or back for all the different allergens they are testing and also do a negative and positive control test. This checks that your body is not overreacting or suppressed by medication. You will usually be asked to stop taking antihistamines up to five days before your tests so they do not affect the results.

A small drop of the liquid or the fresh produce is put on your skin and then the skin is pricked briefly with a sharp probe so it can enter the bloodstream. These will then be left for 15-20 minutes to see if the skin reacts. Your allergist will measure the size of the bump and weal, the red area around it, to determine how much you reacted. A weal of 3mm diameter is generally considered a positive reaction. The larger the weal, the more likely you are to be allergic to that substance but this cannot predict the severity of a reaction.

A small amount of steroid cream will help ease any itching and the weals should disappear within an hour. Rarely, skin prick tests can cause more severe reactions and these will be treated immediately in the clinic.

Patch tests

Patch tests are used to see whether you are allergic to particular chemicals or substances and are often used to identify causes of skin allergies. The allergens are applied to your back and left on for up to 48 hours to check for any reactions.

Blood tests

Blood tests, also known as RAST (radioallergosorbent) tests, can be a good way to test for multiple different allergies at one time and show the amount of IgE antibodies your body produces to certain substances.

The blood will need to be sent to the lab for analysis, so it takes longer to get the results and they are more expensive to perform, so skin prick tests are usually the first choice. However, blood tests may be done if skin prick tests are not available and this is often the case in regional centres where there isn't access to a specialised allergy clinic. Blood tests are also good if the skin is too sensitive or covered in eczema, or if people cannot stop taking antihistamine. They may also be used if a solution for a specific allergen is not available or if someone has had such a severe reaction in the past, skin prick tests are considered too dangerous.

Different scales are used to report the results of RAST tests (see: table 4) but the higher the levels, the more likely someone is to have an allergic reaction. Although like the skin prick tests, it cannot necessarily predict the severity of a reaction. Many people will often have slightly elevated IgE levels if they suffer from asthma and eczema, so a low positive may not indicate a true allergy. They should always be interpreted alongside a medical history.

Test results

Unfortunately, it is not as simple as a positive result indicating an allergy and a negative result meaning you don't have one. Allergy tests can often produce 'false positives', meaning your results are positive for a food or substance you actually have no problem with. This may be because your body is sensitised to it but does not react, or the test is picking up proteins that cross react with other similar substances – such as someone who is peanut allergic reacting to other legumes or someone with birch pollen allergy reacting to hazelnut. It is also possible to have a 'false negative', where the test is not showing an allergy you know you react to, although this is less common. This is why it is important for any tests to be interpreted by a trained allergist who can also take into account a patient's previous reactions and medical history.

Endoscopy and biopsy

Some allergic conditions like Eosinophilic Gastrointestinal Disease (EGID) can only be diagnosed by looking inside the gastrointestinal tract. This is done by endoscopy when a small tube (endoscope) with a light and camera on it is passed through the tract. This can also be used to perform a biopsy, where a small tissue sample is taken so it can be analysed further.

Component tests

Many foods contain a number of different proteins and component tests are able to narrow down exactly which ones someone is reacting to. This can be helpful to predict cross reactivity with other foods as well as the risk and likely severity of a reaction. Component tests are relatively new and not widely used in the UK currently but they do offer potential for building a more accurate picture of someone's allergy profile.

Dietician

If you have food allergies, you should be referred to a dietician who will help make sure you or your child are eating a healthy, balanced diet. They will ask you lots of questions about your daily meals and food intake. If you have already had allergy tests and been told to avoid certain foods, they can offer alternative sources of nutrients and are also able to advise about baby and infant formulas and milk replacements.

If you have non-IgE reactions, then tests will be unable to diagnose your allergies and a dietician can support you with an elimination diet. They will also support anyone who is attempting reintroduction and can provide a step by step plan as well as recipes and suggestions of foods to try.

(see more: chapter 16)

Food or drug challenges

Allergy tests can help predict the likelihood of an allergic reaction, but they are not completely reliable and the only way to be sure is to carry out a challenge. This may be suggested if tests are inconclusive. Your doctor may also suggest a challenge if your test results have decreased over time, or if there is a possibility you may be able to introduce some levels of food. For example, many people can tolerate baked egg or milk in cakes and biscuits who cannot tolerate it more lightly cooked in an omelette or boiled egg.

Sometimes, if you have been diagnosed as a child but not had any serious reactions for a long time, it can be a good idea to have a food challenge to see if you can reintroduce things into your diet.

Challenges should only be carried out at the hospital or allergy clinic when you are in good health and any asthma is well controlled. They are safe and severe reactions are rare, but staff will monitor you closely and have medication close by in case it is needed.

You will usually be asked to attend the hospital in the morning and should expect to be there for most the day. The doctor will check that you are well and may repeat any skin prick tests. You will then be given small amounts of the allergen in incremental doses, monitored closely.

In the case of foods, you will first have the allergen rubbed on your skin, then your lips before eating a crumb and slowly increasing the doses, waiting around 20 minutes each time to check for a reaction. If you have a clear reaction, the challenge will be stopped. Once the challenge has been completed, you will need to wait for another few hours to check for reactions. If you have any further reactions once you leave the clinic, you should avoid the food and contact your allergist.

'Reassure your child by chatting about the challenge beforehand, so your little one knows exactly what to expect. Make it clear that they will be trying something they are, or used to be, allergic to and prepare them for the fact a reaction could happen, but also explain that if it does, they will be in the best place possible for it to be dealt with. The last thing you want is for your child to develop a phobia of hospitals and get anxious before their next visit to their allergist. If your child is showing signs of anxiety, ask one of the nurses on the ward whether a play specialist is available. Play specialists are amazing at distracting the children's attention away from the challenge and getting rid of any of the tension that might have accumulated.'   *Mel Knibb*

Care plans

Your doctor should provide you with a detailed care plan outlining what to avoid and what to do if you have a reaction. This will include different treatment for mild or more severe reactions and detail the medication and dose you need to take, as well as how to administer it. Talk this through with them and make sure you fully understand what to do and have the medication in place. They should also show you how to take your medication correctly and how to use an adrenaline auto-injector, if needed. Things to ask or confirm are:

- What substances do I need to avoid? Do I need to avoid them fully?
- What kind of reactions should I expect?
- What do I do if I have a reaction?
- Do I need an adrenaline auto-injector and how do I use it?
- When would you consider a challenge?
- When will I have my next appointment or tests?

You can update the care plan with your personal information and emergency contact details and make sure you have a digital and hard copy. It is a good idea to keep a care plan with your medication and to print off extra copies to give to family, caregivers or your workplace.

> 'It's all too easy to succumb to the worry and fear that comes with being an allergy mum. There's a constant ticking time bomb just waiting to explode as you never know when the next reaction will happen, nor how severe it will be. By taking simple steps such as carrying a full medi pack with you at all times, and teaching and educating those that will be looking after your little one at school how to manage an allergic reaction will help to alleviate some of that worry. You can't live your life as a "what if" and I always live by the moto of "allergies are life changing but they shouldn't be life defining".
> *Nathalie Newman*

Expert Insight: Food challenges

Roisin Fitzsimons
Consultant allergy nurse

At what age do you carry out allergy tests or food challenges?

We can test people at any age and it is important to raise awareness among GPs that we can test young children and babies, to get referrals made earlier. We tend to test young children yearly and then at school age, again before secondary school and at about 14 before we transition them to the adult service. That adolescent age is a tricky one. You're becoming more independent, want to fit in and we look at how to help them.

Why should people take part in food challenges?

A food challenge is the only definitive way to diagnose if someone is actually allergic or not. We are challenging more young children with nut allergies because of the evidence that they might be allergic to one nut but able to tolerate others. We now know that if we can get certain foods into a child's diet when they are very young, we can prevent them from developing an allergy. It is important to know for certain if you need to avoid a food. If you are allergic, we can help you be vigilant and avoid that food. If not, it opens up so many options and improves quality of life to not avoid a food unnecessarily.

What would you say to people worried about having an anaphylactic reaction during a challenge?

A food challenge is a safe procedure, although it is not without its risks. The nurses who perform food challenges are experts in the procedure and have extensive knowledge and experience. The factor which poses a risk of having a more severe reaction (anaphylaxis) is illness and in particular a worsening of asthma. Therefore, before a food challenge begins, you or your child will be assessed to ensure they are well enough to perform the challenge. It is a safe procedure and we have a very low number of anaphylactic reactions. The team know what signs to look out for and signs of a reaction are always identified and treated straight away.

How can people prepare for the experience?

We try to make the experience as friendly and relaxed as possible and create a nice, non-threatening environment. We encourage people to bring in food their children like to hide the allergen they are being tested to – even if it's disgusting. We don't mind feeding them fish hidden in a jam sandwich! Older children and adults may remember having a reaction and we want to give as much reassurance as possible. Preparation is key and we try to find the right balance between enough information so they know what's going on, but not too much. We support the parents too, as kids pick up on what they are feeling. I would encourage parents to find out as much as possible before the challenge, so they know what will happen on the day and afterwards, as it's important if the child isn't allergic to the food that they eat it regularly in their diet. It's important for families that they are prepared and if after reading the information they are given, they still have questions, they should call the allergy service, who will help provide further clarification.

Chapter 7

ANAPHYLAXIS

Anaphylaxis is a severe allergic reaction where chemicals are released into the blood stream, rather than into a localised area. It occurs with IgE-mediated allergies and usually happens within minutes of coming into contact with the allergen but can happen up to a couple of hours later. Anaphylaxis can cause difficulty breathing and a dangerous drop in blood pressure and requires immediate medical attention and treatment with adrenaline (epinephrine).

The most common causes of anaphylactic reactions are foods, drugs and insect stings and, although fatal reactions are rare, up to 20 people in the UK die each year.

Symptoms of anaphylaxis can include:

- Swelling of tongue and/or throat
- Difficulty in swallowing or speaking
- Persistent cough
- Stridor – a high pitched wheezing sound
- Difficulty breathing
- Severe abdominal pain or repeated vomiting
- Weakness, dizziness or collapse
- Feeling of impending doom

Symptoms may start off mildly, with a rash or itching for example, and progress into anaphylaxis or severe symptoms may be present from the onset without any of the typical mild ones like hives.

A number of factors can influence the severity of an allergic reaction including uncontrolled asthma, the amount of allergen ingested, illness, heat or exercise.

'It is terrifying watching your child go through anaphylaxis, not knowing if the medicine will work. I have stayed calm when it's happened but have reacted afterwards with a lot of tears! I found myself cancelling social engagements and avoiding invites to Sunday lunches, coffees etc. It becomes isolating. I've been clearer about my boundaries and now I explain politely and clearly why things need to be the way they are. That has helped keep my son safe which in turn calms me down. Friends put me in touch with their friends who have allergic children and has helped too as I felt less alone with it all.'   *Ellie Ludlam*

Who it at risk?

Unfortunately, tests cannot predict the severity of a reaction, only the likelihood of one happening and it is also not possible to predict how severe a reaction will be based on a previous one. You are more at risk of an anaphylactic reaction if you:

- Have had one beforehand
- Have severe or uncontrolled asthma
- React strongly to small amounts of an allergen
- Have contact reactions

There are tests available which look at different components of allergens and which proteins people react to. This can give a more accurate picture, but they are not readily used.

Idiopathic anaphylaxis

Sometimes, even after tests and investigations, doctors may be unable to find the cause for an anaphylactic reaction. It is then called idiopathic. There may still be an external trigger, but it has not been found, or it might be the body's immune system working in overdrive. Often the immune system settles on its own, but your doctor may prescribe treatment such as oral steroids to try and control it.

Exercise induced anaphylaxis

Exercise induced anaphylaxis is rare and is when an anaphylactic reaction happens after physical activity. It may occur alone or be triggered in combination with eating a certain food beforehand. Wheat is often found as the trigger, although other foods have also been reported and there have also been cases where the cold has contributed to a reaction.

Treating an anaphylactic reaction

Most allergic reactions can be treated with antihistamines or will subside on their own but the only first line treatment for an anaphylactic reaction is adrenaline (epinephrine). This is the only drug which can stop the cells releasing further chemicals and reduce the swelling, open airways and raise blood pressure. People at risk of an anaphylactic reaction should carry adrenaline auto-injectors at all times. The quicker they are used, the more likely they are to be effective. If someone has an anaphylactic reaction you should:

- Administer adrenaline
- Call 999
- Lie them down and do not move them
- Raise their shoulders or sit them up if they are having trouble breathing
- Administer second dose after 5 minutes in the other leg if symptoms persist
- Try and note what caused the reaction and when adrenaline was administered

In most cases, adrenaline works quickly, symptoms subside and there is no need for further treatment. However, it is important to always call an ambulance and go to hospital. Adrenaline wears off and it may be necessary to administer more or to receive further treatment including antihistamines, steroids or oxygen. You should also be monitored for up to 4-6 hours in case of a biphasic reaction, where symptoms subside but reoccur hours later. It is possible for biphasic reactions to happen up to 72 hours later, but this is rare.

Many people are worried about how they will know if they should administer adrenaline. Your doctor should give you a clear care plan to follow but if you are in doubt, then it is better to administer it. Adrenaline will cause a faster heartbeat but there are no major adverse side effects, whereas the consequences of not using it can be fatal.

If someone suffers an anaphylactic reaction and you do not have access to an adrenaline auto-injector, administer antihistamine and any inhaler, lie them down and keep them still, and call an ambulance immediately.

Recovery

After an anaphylactic reaction, you may feel weak, tired and sore and need time for your body to fully recover. You may be given a course of steroids to help reduce any inflammation.

It is also natural to feel overwhelmed and emotional about the experience as the psychological effects can be difficult to cope with (see: chapter 15).

If your child suffered anaphylaxis, take time to reassure them, talk about what happened and help them process their fears. It is also tough on the parents so treat yourself gently and reach out for support from friends, family, your GP or online groups.

In hospital

It may seem strange to worry about anaphylaxis when you are in hospital but medical settings, including dentists, can present lots of risks. Be sure to communicate any drug allergies, make sure it is clearly labelled on your records and wear a hospital band to alert all staff. The same is true if you have a latex allergy when dressings, plasters or gloves may be an issue.

Food allergies can also be a problem as unfortunately, many hospital caterers are not well informed, nor do they have strict procedures in place. Ask for your food allergies to be clearly labelled at your bed and on your records. Talk to the caterers, double check each meal or take your own safe food if possible.

Chapter 8

ALLERGY MEDICATION

The first line treatment for most allergies is avoiding the trigger but there are a number of medications that can help prevent, control or treat reactions. These can improve people's quality of life and in some cases, be life-saving. Talk to your doctor about your treatment options and any side effects.

Antihistamines

Most allergic reactions can be treated, or prevented, with antihistamines, which work by blocking histamine receptors and stopping it being released into the body. They are most commonly used in liquid or tablet form but can also be ingredients in lotions, eye drops and nasal sprays. There are types that may make you feel sleepy like chlorphenamine – often know by the brand name Piriton, and non-drowsy ones, like cetirizine or loratadine. Your doctor will be able to advise which is best for you. You may take them just to treat an acute allergic reaction, or as a daily dose to help prevent symptoms, sometimes just at certain times of year – for example, during pollen season.

Adrenaline auto-injectors

If you are at risk of an anaphylactic reaction, then your doctor should prescribe you adrenaline auto-injectors – often referred to as an adrenaline pen or by the common brand name EpiPen – which you need to carry at all times. These contain a dose of adrenaline that can be administered through a one-time use needle injected into the outer thigh in an emergency situation.

The dose you require will differ depending on age and weight and will be prescribed by your doctor. You should be shown how to use them correctly and provided with trainer pens, so you and any caregivers can practice. There are different types of adrenaline auto-injector available in the UK – EpiPen, Jext and Emerade. They all do the same thing but are operated slightly differently, so make sure you are aware of which one you have been given and are confident in using it.

Adrenaline auto-injectors can be affected by extremes of temperature, so it is important to keep them out of direct sunlight, very cold conditions and not leave them in the car overnight. You may want to buy an insulated case to help with this. All adrenaline auto-injectors have an expiry date so make a note of this and get a repeat prescription in plenty of time. All three manufacturers run an expiry alert service which you can sign up to. You need to dispose of them in a sharps container, which you can obtain from your doctor or pharmacist.

In most cases, an allergist will prescribe you an adrenaline auto-injector if you need one, but GPs are also able to do so if they believe you are at risk. The need will be assessed on an individual basis and the 2016 guidelines from the British Society for Allergy and Clinical Immunology (BSACI) advise that someone should be given an adrenaline auto-injector if they:

- have suffered an anaphylactic reaction where the cause is unknown (idiopathic anaphylaxis)
- have suffered an anaphylactic reaction where the allergen cannot easily be avoided
- had a reaction to trace amounts of the allergen
- suffer food-dependant exercise-induced anaphylaxis
- have significant other risk factors e.g. asthma in someone with food allergy
- are allergic to high-risk allergens, for example nuts, and have another risk factor, even if the reaction was relatively mild

The guidelines also suggest that people at low risk may only need to carry one adrenaline auto-injector. However, the Medicines and Healthcare Products Regulatory Agency (MHRA) advised in 2014, and again in 2017, that people at risk of anaphylaxis should carry two auto-injectors at all times. This is in case one fails to work or is delivered incorrectly, if a second dose is needed in a severe reaction or if there is a delay in reaching hospital and the reaction progresses. This view is supported by the European Medicines Agency (EMA), Allergy UK and Anaphylaxis Campaign.

If you have trouble being prescribed adrenaline auto-injectors or are only being offered one, then take a copy of the MHRA guidelines (see: resources) to your GP.

You should also be prescribed additional auto-injectors to leave at primary school or nursery as these will usually need to be stored onsite. Since October 2017, schools are also able to purchase adrenaline auto-injectors, without a prescription, to store and use on children who are at a known risk of anaphylaxis if their own pens are not working or not available. (see: resources)

Emollients and wet wraps

Emollients, or quality moisturisers, are the first line treatment for eczema as good hydration helps repair the skin barrier. Mild eczema can usually be managed with over-the-counter emollients but there are a range available on prescription and you may need to test a few to see which works best.

Some people, especially children, may benefit from scratch sleeves, long sleeved clothing made of natural fibres which help them not to scratch inflamed skin. Wet wraps may also be used, when tubular bandages are soaked in water and layered with emollient to help trap moisture in.

Corticosteroids (steroids)

Steroids are not used to directly stop an allergic reaction but treat one of the common symptoms, inflammation. They are often given after an acute allergic reaction to help calm the immune system. They are also used in the treatment of eczema and asthma. Topical steroids, like hydrocortisone, are used when eczema cannot be controlled through emollients. Oral steroids, like prednisone, are used to treat inflammation in the lungs, while nasal sprays and eye drops containing steroids can also be used to treat allergic rhinitis.

Inhalers

There are two types of inhalers used to treat asthma and respiratory symptoms. The first are preventative steroid inhalers (e.g. Clenil). These need to be taken daily and are an important treatment for keeping asthma under control and preventing any attacks by reducing swelling and inflammation. People are often concerned about taking daily steroids but the dose in inhalers is very low and presents no ill-effects for long term use.

The others are reliever inhalers (e.g. Ventolin) which help open up the airways by relaxing the muscles when they are tightening. Your doctor should show you how to take these effectively and provide you with a spacer, a plastic tube with a mask on, to help you administer them to children. Up to 70 per cent of people are not taking inhalers correctly[1] During an asthma attack, a nebuliser may be used by doctors or paramedics to deliver a fine mist of medication through a mask, often alongside oxygen.

Anti-leukotrienes

Leukotrienes are chemical compounds that help protect the body but when they are triggered by allergies they can cause inflammation in the airways. Anti-leukotrienes help block this process. The most commonly used is Montelaukast which can be taken by adults or children in tablet or powder form to help control asthma and seasonal allergies.

Anti-IgE therapy

Anti-IgE therapy works by blocking immunoglobulin E (IgE) antibodies which trigger inflammation and allergic reactions. These drugs, the most common being Omalizumab, are given by injection every 2-4 weeks and are currently used to treat severe allergic asthma that is not responding to regular inhaled steroids. They can also be used to treat chronic urticaria.

Calcineurin inhibitors

Calcineurin inhibitors help block a chemical called calcineurin which activates inflammation in the skin. They can be used to treat atopic eczema if emollients and steroid creams are not working, as well as other inflammatory skin conditions.

Alternative therapies

There are lots of practitioners who claim to be able to treat or cure allergies with alternative therapies, homeopathy, Chinese medicine or probiotics. Some treatments address the symptoms of allergies, while others work on reducing inflammation in the body and rebalancing the immune system and microbiome.

There is a growing body of research looking into these areas but there is currently no medical evidence that they can treat or cure the body's immune response. Talk to your doctor about any additional treatment you are seeking and discuss an integrative approach to be sure it does not pose a risk or interfere with your prescribed medication.

Immunotherapy

Immunotherapy involves slowly introducing small amounts of an allergen into the body and gradually increasing the dose. This helps the immune system become less sensitive and reduces the symptoms the next time the body encounters it. It is not a cure for allergies but can help improve quality of life and decrease the risk of anaphylaxis.

There are a number of different types of immunotherapy:

Subcutaneous immunotherapy (SCIT)

Subcutaneous immunotherapy involves a small amount of allergen being given by injection, usually at different intervals over three years.

Sublingual immunotherapy (SLIT)

Sublingual immunotherapy can be used instead of SCIT and involves the allergen being placed under the tongue to dissolve, usually in the form of a small tablet. These need to be taken daily at home, usually also for three years.

SCIT and SLIT immunotherapy are currently available in the UK for tree and grass pollens, dust mites, and animal or venom allergies. This treatment is considered by doctors if someone is still showing severe symptoms even after taking all other medication correctly, or if someone needs it to do their job. Itching and mild swelling are common side effects and patients may have some flu-like symptoms but serious reactions are rare.

Oral immunotherapy

Oral immunotherapy is used for food allergies. Participants start by eating an extremely small amount of the food protein – for example, a powdered fraction of a peanut – which is then very slowly and carefully increased until patients are tolerating a standard amount, for example, around six peanuts in one sitting. The first dose and any increases will be given in hospital and then regular doses of a set amount are continued at home.

Participants need to continue to strictly eat the maintenance dose in their diets at set intervals to remain desensitised to the food, even after the treatment programme has finished. Small scale studies show up to 80 per cent of people taking part in oral immunotherapy become desensitised.[2] There are potential side effects and many people suffer gastrointestinal symptoms or mild allergic reactions during treatment, but cases of anaphylaxis are rare. Reactions usually happen during the initial stages or when a dose is increased and very rarely during the maintenance doses taken at home.

It is still unknown whether immunotherapies will be able to lead from desensitisation to tolerance, where people continue not to react to the allergen even when no longer eating regular doses. There have been some studies which show patients have been able to stop maintenance doses for 1-2 months and still remain desensitised but there has been no evidence yet of long term tolerance.

The only oral immunotherapy currently available in the UK is for peanuts, at a private clinic at Addenbrookes hospital in Cambridgeshire. The programme is for 7-16-year olds after an initial assessment to see if they are suitable, taking into account previous reactions, other allergies and asthma. A clinical trial is also being carried out at Guy's Hospital to see if a similar immunotherapy would be effective for adults.

In other countries, such as America, oral immunotherapy is more widely available and is used to treat many other food allergies including tree nuts, sesame, milk and egg. It is still relatively new and opinions on its effectiveness and risks vary.

Oral immunotherapy must be carried out by a trained medical professional and participants need to stick to a strict protocol of doses. This is not something that you should attempt to replicate at home. New immunotherapies, including a pill and a patch, are being trialled and it is an area of allergy management that will likely develop and become more accessible in coming years. Ask your allergist about upcoming trials you or your child may be eligible for.

Chapter 9

ALLERGIES IN INFANTS

Allergies are on the rise and are usually first seen in infants, so it is a challenge that many parents have to face. It can be distressing to see your child in pain and unfortunately, it can be difficult to get the right support and diagnosis.

Cow's milk allergy

The most common food allergy in infants is cow's milk protein allergy, affecting up to 7 per cent of children under one.[1] It is usually the first one to present itself, either when an infant is given a formula containing cow's milk or because they are reacting from cow's milk proteins via the breastmilk. It is a complex allergy with different presentations that can make the diagnosis a challenge.

Cow's milk allergy can be IgE-mediated (immediate), non IgE (delayed) or a combination of both. The most common type of cow's milk allergy is non-IgE-mediated where delayed symptoms are observed several hours or days after a feed such as severe abdominal discomfort, colic or reflux, frequent discoloured or frothy stools, with mucus or streaks of blood in them, or eczema. Immediate IgE-mediated reactions – which are more common when using formula – can display hives, swelling of eyes/lips/face, vomiting or difficulty breathing. It is important that an early and accurate diagnosis is made, specifically for the IgE-mediated allergy due to the risk of an anaphylactic reaction.

Other food allergies

Many infants with a non-IgE-mediated cow's milk allergy may also react to soya as the proteins in these foods are very similar. It is also possible that some highly sensitive infants may also react to other food proteins through their mothers' breastmilk. Although most reactions are from common food groups including cow's milk, egg, peanut, sesame, soya, shellfish, fish or tree nuts, it is possible to be allergic to any food and it can become difficult to pinpoint the cause accurately.

Infant eczema

In 45 per cent of children with eczema, it develops before they are one and about half of those with early onset eczema (starting in the first few months) will show an allergic sensitisation by the time they are two.[2] Eczema can often be dismissed as a mild condition, but it can seriously affect quality of life, especially for infants and their parents. It is difficult to stop young children from scratching and it often leads to disturbed sleep and exhaustion.

There is a leading theory that babies develop allergies when they are exposed to food proteins through their skin, especially when the skin barrier is broken like in eczema. This makes it particularly important to try and get eczema under control as soon as possible.

Emollients (moisturisers) are the main treatment for dry skin conditions like eczema. Emollients should be applied generously and several times a day. Always make sure you wash your hands before applying them to prevent spreading bacteria and apply them using gentle, downward smooth strokes. Try to use a pump or tube as tubs can become easily contaminated from hands Bathing is good for eczema skin but water alone can be very drying so adding an emollient oil or ointment to the bath will help. As heat is a common trigger of eczema, keep the water temperature tepid and pat instead of rub dry to avoid damaging the skin further. Also, stick to a mild and sensitive washing detergent and all natural fibres like cotton for your child's clothing, avoiding wool as this can cause a 'prickle' sensation.

If the frequent and generous use of emollients alone is not keeping the eczema under control and it has become flared, then a steroid cream or ointment may be needed and your GP will be able to prescribe this,

For any eczema that is persistent and uncontrolled by these methods, you may need a referral to a dermatologist or paediatric allergist.

Environmental allergies or viral wheeze

If your child has a persisting blocked 'snuffly nose' which is constantly congested, has 'allergy shiners' (dark circles under the eyes caused by sinus congestion) or suffers a persistent cough or wheeze then you may want to consider environmental allergies such as pets, house dust mites, mould or pollen as a cause. These may also be exacerbating any eczema. Sometimes, a wheeze or cough that comes and goes may be caused by a virus. These symptoms can develop into asthma, but this is rarely diagnosed in children under five as many grow out of it as their airways develop.

Getting a diagnosis

Symptoms similar to a food allergy can be seen in other common childhood conditions including eczema, colic and reflux, or being unsettled and crying. Unfortunately, health professionals may try to treat these individual symptoms rather than look at the overall picture. Many parents have numerous trips to the doctor and it can be very disheartening trying to get the help you need. Remember that you know your child best. Arm yourself with all the information – NICE and iMAP guidelines (see: resources) – and push for the support you need. Discuss concerns with your GP, but you will come to know your child well so if you feel that your GP is not listening then see a different one (for a second opinion) or talk to your health visitor who may also be able to help. If your child is showing any severe symptoms or you are worried about their immediate health, take them directly to your local A&E or call an ambulance.

> 'Although I have allergies, it has been a big learning curve and I discovered that as a parent you know your child the best and know if something is wrong. I found lots of health care professionals didn't take my concerns very seriously and also that lots of doctors don't have the knowledge I would expect them to have about allergies. I would say to anyone who suspects an allergy to write it all down and to be persistent with health care professionals and to keep going and raising your concerns. I also took photographs of reactions to show health care professionals so they can see for themselves. It can be a frustrating road ahead but keep going.'
> *Amy Wobbaka*

Breastfeeding

Earlier advice to avoid common high-risk food allergens during pregnancy and breastfeeding has been dismissed and mothers are now encouraged to eat a wide and healthy diet. Unless you have a food allergy or baby is showing obvious symptoms to a food passing through your breastmilk then you should continue to eat normally, even if you have another child with allergies.

Breastfeeding is beneficial to mother and baby and can play a part in preventing allergies by strengthening your child's healthy gut bacteria and microbiome. The World Health Organisation encourages exclusive breastfeeding until 6 months followed by continued breastfeeding alongside food until 2 years old.

It is commonly misperceived that babies cannot react to allergens through breastmilk, but this is not true. The amount of protein that passes via breastmilk is very small, but babies can still have IgE-mediated (immediate) and non-IgE (delayed) reactions to it. It can be very discouraging to feel you are causing your baby harm through foods you are eating but many people are able to continue breastfeeding by cutting out the suspected food allergen(s) from their diet. You need to make sure you are still eating a balanced healthy diet that is providing you and your baby with enough nutrition. If you are thinking about cutting foods out, always consult a doctor or dietician who can support you.

If cow's milk allergy is suspected, this will need to be eliminated from the breastfeeding mother's diet in all forms. Other mammalian milks (sheep, goat, buffalo) also contain similar proteins so should be avoided too. This can be really daunting to begin with, but the good news is that there are lots of dairy-free plant-based alternatives available and many online support groups. (see: resources)

You will need to cut it out for 2-4 weeks to let it fully clear out of your system and confirm an allergy but you may see a change in your baby much quicker than that. You should take a calcium and vitamin D supplement to maintain your own health while doing this.

If you feel your baby is still showing symptoms, then the next likely allergens are soy, egg and wheat. Consult your doctor or dietician about cutting each of these out individually so you can see if it makes a difference. Unfortunately, it can be really difficult to know exactly what your baby is reacting to and can feel like a puzzle you cannot solve. It can be worth keeping a diary of what you have eaten and your baby's symptoms to see if you can identify a pattern. However, there are lots of factors like illness and teething that may affect this.

If your baby is still showing symptoms once you have removed the common food allergens, is continuing to lose weight, or if you are struggling mentally or physically with the restricted diet, you may want to consider moving on to formula.

"Breastfeeding with allergies can feel incredibly daunting at the beginning. The overwhelming pressure knowing if you eat anything you shouldn't, you will be poisoning your own child. But this feeling is hugely outweighed by the milk smiles, smell of their delicious head and the incredible change your will see in your little one once they are allergen free. Seeing how much happier and healthier they are will absolutely drive you to continue doing what you're doing and as with everything, I promise if does get much, much easier. Be strong enough to ensure what you're eating is safe and strong in the knowledge you're doing the very best for your little one."   *Lauren Gordon*

Prescription and non-dairy milks

There are a number of cow's milk-free formula milks available and if your baby has reacted to regular formula, or you suspect an allergy and are moving on from breastfeeding, then talk to your doctor. Many cow's milk-free formulas are available on prescription and it will depend on your child's reactions as to which one is most appropriate.

Hypoallergenic (low allergen) formulas still contain cow's milk proteins but they have been extensively hydrolysed, or broken down, so the immune system is more likely to tolerate them. This type of formula is safe and will relieve symptoms for most infants with cow's milk allergy. Amino acid formulas are used when infants are still reacting to extensively hydrolysed formulas or if a baby has had a severe reaction to cow's milk or multiple allergies. Amino acid formulas do not contain any cow's milk proteins.

It can be a bit of trial and error finding the right formula. If you think your baby is still reacting, go back to the GP and ask to try another one. Some GPs will not want to prescribe an amino acid-based formula without a referral from a dietician or allergy specialist. However, this can take time and the iMap guidelines (see: resources) state your GP should consider a prescription formula while still waiting for a specialist appointment.

Soy formulas

If your baby reacts to cow's milk but not to soy, then you may be able to use a soy based formula if they are over 6 months old. These are not suitable for infants under 6 months, due to the large amount of phytoestrogens in them which may disrupt their hormonal development. Talk to a dietician about whether you are able to switch to a soy formula alongside weaning.

Dairy free milk alternatives

After breastfeeding or bottle feeding on a nutritionally complete formula, you can begin to introduce solids around 6 months alongside your baby's milk when they can hold their head up unaided and are developmentally ready. At this age, regular dairy free milk alternatives can be used in cooking and baking.

There are lots of dairy-free plant-based milks available including soy, oat, almond, coconut, rice and hemp. It is important to talk to a dietician about the best one for your child's needs. As long as you choose a fortified one, then they have the required amount of calcium in them along with other nutrients such as vitamin D. NICE guidelines recommend they are not used as a main milk source until after 2 years of age and rice milk is not recommended as a main drink for children under 5 because of high levels of arsenic.

Weaning

Weaning a baby can be daunting if you know or suspect they have food allergies and every new food can be filled with worry. However, there are lots of steps you can take to make it go as smoothly as possible and minimise the risks.

If symptoms of an IgE-mediated food allergy occur, then your GP should make a referral for assessment and allergy testing, although because of the difficulties with accessing services and waiting times, it can be difficult to get a referral before you start weaning. If your child suffers an immediate reaction during weaning, stop that food immediately, treat any symptoms and do not delay in seeking immediate medical help.

Keep yourself a notebook to record all the foods you feed your baby and any reactions. This will help you feel more in control of the situation and may help to identify any patterns for delayed reactions. Introduce new foods when your baby is well and is able to be observed for the duration of the day. Each new food should be introduced one at a time every three days. Start off with the least allergenic foods – things like sweet potato, carrot, apple – and introduce them well cooked first as they are less likely to cause a reaction. If your baby has had a previous reaction to a food, don't reintroduce it until you have had medical advice. If you are anxious about new foods, then each time you introduce one, rub a small amount on their lip, followed by a small crumb or taste before a full spoonful or bite. Leave 20 minutes between each of these stages to watch for any immediate symptoms. Following these steps will help you watch out and react to any adverse effects.

Recent research suggests that the previous advice to delay introducing the most allergenic foods, including peanuts, may be contributing the development of food allergies, rather than preventing them. (see more: chapter 17)

'Starting out on our allergy free weaning journey was an exciting and apprehensive time- preparation, having a plan and taking it at baby's pace was key to helping keep Henry safe. We began weaning trying one fruit/vegetable at a time for around 3-5 days. We would note down the food, how much food was consumed, any reactions along with the symptoms. Keeping a "food diary" became a key tool for us in those early weaning months - it enabled us to keep a comprehensive account of Henry's "safe foods" and feel confident at a time which can be daunting for most parents of allergy babies.'   *Rachael Egginton*

Vaccinations

Many people dealing with allergies are wary about giving their children vaccinations as there have been mixed messages about whether they are safe or could even cause food allergies. There is no evidence that vaccines cause allergies and they are generally safe for food allergic children, although it is possible to react to the individual ingredients.

The flu vaccination and nasal flu spray, introduced in 2013 for children, both contain small amounts of residual egg protein, so it was previously uncertain whether they were safe to give to people with egg allergies. While it was concluded that the regular vaccine contained too little egg protein to cause a reaction, researchers carried out a study into the safety of the nasal spray.

The Sniffle Study showed no anaphylactic reactions in any of the 282 children who received the spray, many of whom had previous anaphylaxis to egg or a history of asthma. A few children had minor reactions or coughing and wheezing within three days. The current guidance is that it is safe for all children with an egg allergy to receive the flu vaccine. However, for precaution, if your child has had an admission to intensive care as a result of a severe allergic reaction to egg you should discuss it with your doctor or allergy specialist.

Playgroups

The thought of taking your child to a play group or soft play when they have allergies can be stressful. If they suffer from eczema, you may worry about people staring or what others may say.

Many parents have been in this situation and one of the benefits of allergies increasing is that more people are aware of them. Try to find one place to go that you feel comfortable with. This may be a playgroup that does not serve food, or somewhere that is welcoming and where you feel able to talk.

It can be best to address the issues clearly with the organisers and talk about your child's allergies and what risks there are. Could they limit food and drink to a specific room or section? Could they ask people not to bring snacks for their children and only serve safe ones? Could they have wipes available, so everyone can clean their hands?

Discuss any activities like playdough or crafts using materials like used food containers, balloons, or latex gloves that could be a concern. Many playgroups are very willing to help, especially if you are able to give them some simple steps to make things safer.

Soft play and parks

Soft play can also be difficult as most places serve food alongside the play area and parks are full of people eating, or difficult for grass and pollen allergies. There are some steps you can take to minimise any problems.

- Try to go early in the day when the area may be most clean or less busy
- Visit parks on days when pollen counts are low or after it has rained which will help clear the air
- Put your child in trousers and long-sleeved clothes to avoid contact with allergens
- Always wash your child's hands before they eat

Educating friends and family

Although family should be the easiest group of people to deal with, it is often difficult as it feels more personal if they are not being as supportive as possible. Try not to let emotions run high and work on building a long-term understanding.

Spend time educating your family about allergies so they properly understand what the risks are and how to avoid them. It is also important that they recognise the symptoms. You may want to talk them through your care plan and show them how to administer medication or help them find some resources to read.

Be clear about exactly what you need and offer to help so they do not feel overburdened or confused. You can then look for solutions together by offering safe recipes, a different activity or allergy friendly venue. You may find it easier to host family gatherings, so you can have more control over things, especially until they get used to handling things or you feel more confident that they understand.

Know they want to keep your child safe too, but they will probably make mistakes, buy the wrong things or forget the rules as they don't deal with it every day. Take a deep breath, explain it again and remember it's not because they don't care.

'One of the hardest things to navigate once you have allergies in your life is helping people around you understand them! When my daughter was diagnosed we took her grandparents to the allergist appointment where they learnt some facts and also received training for autoinjector use. I have talked the rest of family and friends through our care plan and also helped them get to grips with autoinjector use by using out of date pens on oranges. If someone doesn't live with allergies then nothing about it is obvious, you need to be thorough in your explanation and show practical tips for dealing with allergies.'   *Clare Hussein*

Expert Advice: Allergies in infants

Dr Adam Fox
Consultant Children's Allergist and Clinical Lead
Evelina London, Guys and St Thomas Trust

What is your experience of allergies being properly recognised in primary care?

When we started the clinic at St Thomas in 2006 we set up an open access email and every day I was getting horrendous stories from parents who just weren't getting enough help. Things have improved and these stories seem much less common now but there are still big gaps in primary care. As a general recommendation, when parents are worried that their child may have a food allergy, I suggest they get a copy of the parents' guide for the NICE food allergy guidance which tells them what to look for, what to ask their GP, what their rights are and what their expectations for care should be. If they are worried about milk allergy, there is a useful resource on the Allergy UK website as part of the iMAP guidelines. Unfortunately, it still can come down to speaking up if you don't feel you're getting what you need.

What link is there between infant eczema and developing allergies?

The worse the eczema is and the earlier it starts, the more likely a child is to develop food allergies. There is now evidence that children may become sensitised to allergens through their skin at a young age. Those with eczema and egg allergies then have a 70-80 per cent chance of developing respiratory allergies or asthma as they grow up.

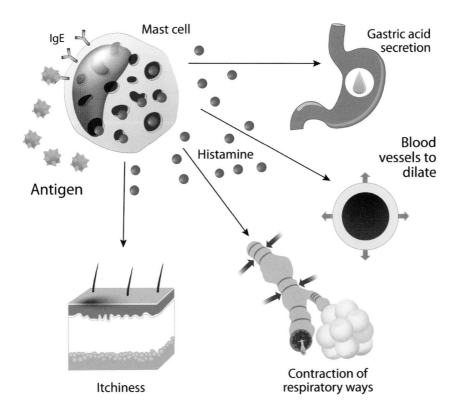

When your body identifies a substance as a threat, cells release histamine to fight it. This can cause a range of reactions from skin rashes and swelling, to breathing difficulties and a dangerous drop in blood pressure.

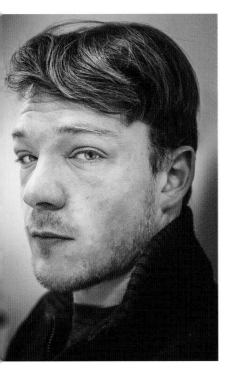

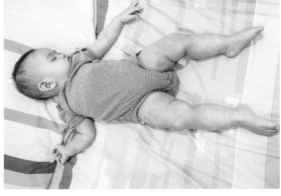

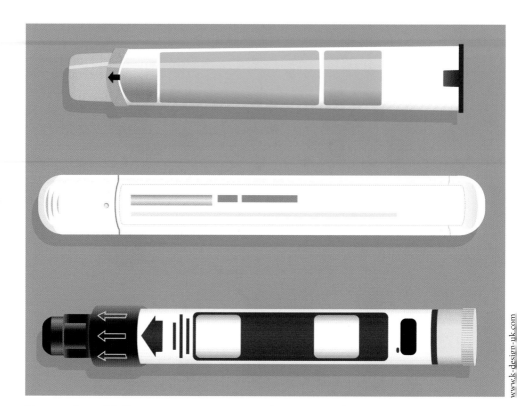

There are lots of different treatment options to manage your allergies, including three type of adrenaline injector. It is important you understand how to use your medication correctly as this can make a big difference to its effectiveness.

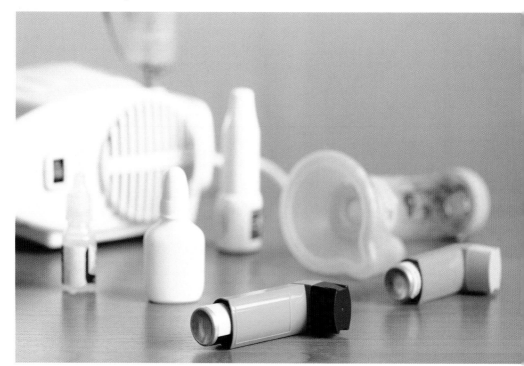

14 Allergens

Food Standards Agency
food.gov.uk

The way allergens are labelled on prepacked foods has changed. The Food Information Regulation, which came into force in December 2014, introduced a requirement that food businesses must provide information about the allergenic ingredients used in any food they sell or provide.

There are 14 major allergens which need to be mentioned (either on a label or through provided information such as menus) when they are used as ingredients in a food. Here are the allergens, and some examples of where they can be found:

1 **Celery**
This includes celery stalks, leaves, seeds and the root called celeriac. You can find celery in celery salt, salads, some meat products, soups and stock cubes.

Cereals containing gluten **2**
Wheat (such as spelt and Khorasan wheat/Kamut), rye, barley and oats is often found in foods containing flour, such as some types of baking powder, batter, breadcrumbs, bread, cakes, couscous, meat products, pasta, pastry, sauces, soups and fried foods which are dusted with flour.

3 **Crustaceans**
Crabs, lobster, prawns and scampi are crustaceans. Shrimp paste, often used in Thai and south-east Asian curries or salads, is an ingredient to look out for.

Eggs **4**
Eggs are often found in cakes, some meat products, mayonnaise, mousses, pasta, quiche, sauces and pastries or foods brushed or glazed with egg.

5 **Fish**
You will find this in some fish sauces, pizzas, relishes, salad dressings, stock cubes and Worcestershire sauce.

Lupin **6**
Yes, lupin is a flower, but it's also found in flour! Lupin flour and seeds can be used in some types of bread, pastries and even in pasta.

7 **Milk**
Milk is a common ingredient in butter, cheese, cream, milk powders and yoghurt. It can also be found in foods brushed or glazed with milk, and in powdered soups and sauces.

Molluscs **8**
These include mussels, land snails, squid and whelks, but can also be commonly found in oyster sauce or as an ingredient in fish stews.

9 **Mustard**
Liquid mustard, mustard powder and mustard seeds fall into this category. This ingredient can also be found in breads, curries, marinades, meat products, salad dressings, sauces and soups.

Nuts **10**
Not to be mistaken with peanuts (which are actually a legume and grow underground), this ingredient refers to nuts which grow on trees, like cashew nuts, almonds and hazelnuts. You can find nuts in breads, biscuits, crackers, desserts, nut powders (often used in Asian curries), stir-fried dishes, ice cream, marzipan (almond paste), nut oils and sauces.

11 **Peanuts**
Peanuts are actually a legume and grow underground, which is why it's sometimes called a groundnut. Peanuts are often used as an ingredient in biscuits, cakes, curries, desserts, sauces (such as satay sauce), as well as in groundnut oil and peanut flour.

Sesame seeds **12**
These seeds can often be found in bread (sprinkled on hamburger buns for example), breadsticks, houmous, sesame oil and tahini. They are sometimes toasted and used in salads.

13 **Soya**
Often found in bean curd, edamame beans, miso paste, textured soya protein, soya flour or tofu, soya is a staple ingredient in oriental food. It can also be found in desserts, ice cream, meat products, sauces and vegetarian products.

Sulphur dioxide (sometimes known as sulphites) **14**
This is an ingredient often used in dried fruit such as raisins, dried apricots and prunes. You might also find it in meat products, soft drinks, vegetables as well as in wine and beer. If you have asthma, you have a higher risk of developing a reaction to sulphur dioxide.

For more information, visit: **food.gov.uk/allergy** or **nhs.uk/conditions/allergies**
Sign up to our allergy alerts on **food.gov.uk/allergy-alerts**, or follow **#AllergyAlert** on Twitter and
Facebook. Let's keep connected at **food.gov.uk/facebook**
Join our conversation **@foodgov**
Watch us on **food.gov.uk/youtube**

The Food Standards Agency recognises 14 top allergens and all food providers have to disclose these ingredients clearly.

allergytravels.com
TRAVEL CHECKLIST

WHEN BOOKING		
Research airline policies		NOTES:
Talk to accommodation supplier about allergies		
Purchase travel insurance		

ONE MONTH TO GO		
Check and renew your medication		NOTES:
Request doctor's letter (if required by airline)		
Update anaphylaxis emergency care/action plan		
Order allergy translation cards		
Gather local information (emergency numbers, hospital locations, etc)		

ONE WEEK TO GO		
Contact airline		BUY SUPPLIES:
Pack extra medication in carry-on luggage		Antibacterial wipes
Research restaurants and call ahead		Medication
NOTES:		Safe snacks
		Other:

ON THE DAY	ON THE PLANE
Talk to ground staff at airport	Tell crew about your allergies
Wear long sleeves or take a blanket to cover your seat	Tell the people around you about your allergy
PACK IN CARRY-ON LUGGAGE:	Make medication easily accessible
Emergency medication	WIPE DOWN:
Anaphylaxis emergency care/action plan	Armrests
Doctor's note	Headrest
Safe snacks	Tray table
Antibacterial wipes	Seatbelt

AT THE DESTINATION		
Visit local supermarket to stock up on safe food		NOTES:
Double check address of accommodation for emergencies		
Show allergy cards to resort chef or restaurants		

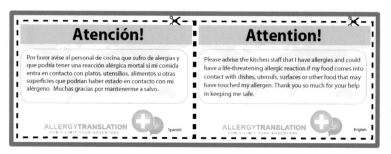

Atención!

Por favor avise al personal de cocina que sufro de alergias y que podría tener una reacción alérgica mortal si mi comida entra en contacto con platos, utensilios, alimentos u otras superficies que podrían haber estado en contacto con mi alérgeno. Muchas gracias por mantenerme a salvo.

ALLERGYTRANSLATION
DON'T LIMIT YOUR ADVENTURE   Spanish

Attention!

Please advise the kitchen staff that I have allergies and could have a life-threatening allergic reaction if my food comes into contact with dishes, utensils, surfaces or other food that may have touched my allergen. Thank you so much for your help in keeping me safe.

ALLERGYTRANSLATION
DON'T LIMIT YOUR ADVENTURE   English

Travelling abroad with allergies takes a little extra work but it can be done safely. Remember to do your research, plan ahead and take an allergy translation card with you.

Allergy Action Plan

THIS CHILD HAS THE FOLLOWING ALLERGIES:

Name:

DOB:

Photo

Emergency contact details:

1)
☎

2)
☎

Child's Weight: ___ Kg

PARENTAL CONSENT: I hereby authorise school staff to administer the medicines listed on this plan, including a 'spare' back-up adrenaline autoinjector (AAI) if available, in accordance with Department of Health guidance on the use of AAIs in schools.

Signed: _____

_____
(PRINT NAME)
Date:

How to give Jext®

1
Form fist around Jext® and PULL OFF YELLOW SAFETY CAP

2
PLACE BLACK END against outer thigh (with or without clothing)

3
PUSH DOWN HARD until a click is heard or felt and hold in place for 10 seconds

4
REMOVE Jext®. Massage injection site for 10 seconds

©The British Society for Allergy & Clinical Immunology, 09/2017

Mild-moderate allergic reaction:
- Swollen lips, face or eyes
- Itchy / tingling mouth
- Hives or itchy skin rash
- Abdominal pain or vomiting
- Sudden change in behaviour

ACTION:
- Stay with the child, call for help if necessary
- Locate adrenaline autoinjector(s)
- Give antihistamine:
- Phone parent/emergency contact   (if vomited, can repeat dose)

Watch for signs of ANAPHYLAXIS
(life-threatening allergic reaction)
Anaphylaxis may occur *without* skin symptoms: **ALWAYS consider anaphylaxis in someone with known food allergy who has** SUDDEN BREATHING DIFFICULTY

AIRWAY: Persistent cough, hoarse voice difficulty swallowing, swollen tongue

BREATHING: Difficult or noisy breathing, wheeze or persistent cough

CONSCIOUSNESS: Persistent dizziness / pale or floppy suddenly sleepy, collapse, unconscious

If ANY ONE (or more) of these signs are present:
1. **Lie child flat:**
   (if breathing is difficult, allow child to sit)
2. **Use Adrenaline autoinjector** (eg. Jext) **without delay**
3. **Dial 999** for ambulance and say ANAPHYLAXIS ("ANA-FIL-AX-IS")

*** IF IN DOUBT, GIVE ADRENALINE ***

After giving Adrenaline:
1. Stay with child until ambulance arrives, **do NOT stand child up**
2. Commence CPR if there are no signs of life
3. Phone parent/emergency contact
4. If no improvement after 5 minutes, **give a 2nd adrenaline dose** using a second autoinjector device, if available.

You can dial 999 from any phone, even if there is no credit left on a mobile. Medical observation in hospital is recommended after anaphylaxis.

Additional instructions:
If wheezy, give adrenaline FIRST, then asthma reliever puffer (blue inhaler) via spacer

This is a medical document that can only be completed by the child's healthcare professional. It must not be altered without their permission. This document provides medical authorisation for schools to administer a 'spare' back-up adrenaline autoinjector if needed, as permitted by the Human Medicines (Amendment) Regulations 2017.

This plan has been prepared by:

SIGN & PRINT NAME: _____

Hospital/Clinic: _____

☎   Date:

www.k-design-uk.com

The best way to take control of your allergies is to be informed, educate others and have a clear action plan. If you have been prescribed adrenaline auto-injectors then make sure you carry two at all times.

We are Allergy Aware!

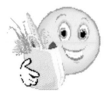

Are you?

Some children have life threatening food allergies. To make sure they can play freely and safely we always:

- Keep food & drink separate to play

- Clean hands after eating

- Clear up crumbs and spills

- Serve inclusive snacks

- Choose food-free activities

- Ask before feeding other children

Please help us follow these simple steps

Thankyou!

There are lots of simple steps other people can take to help keep your child safe whether it is at a playgroup or school. Work together on an allergy management plan to ensure them safe and included.

THE iMAP MILK LADDER

To be used only in children with Mild to Moderate Non-IgE Cow's Milk Allergy
Under the supervision of a healthcare professional
PLEASE SEE THE ACCOMPANYING RECIPE INFORMATION

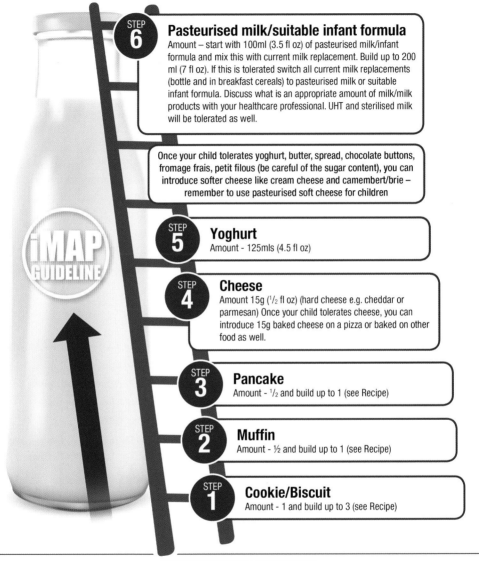

STEP 6 **Pasteurised milk/suitable infant formula**
Amount – start with 100ml (3.5 fl oz) of pasteurised milk/infant formula and mix this with current milk replacement. Build up to 200 ml (7 fl oz). If this is tolerated switch all current milk replacements (bottle and in breakfast cereals) to pasteurised milk or suitable infant formula. Discuss what is an appropriate amount of milk/milk products with your healthcare professional. UHT and sterilised milk will be tolerated as well.

Once your child tolerates yoghurt, butter, spread, chocolate buttons, fromage frais, petit filous (be careful of the sugar content), you can introduce softer cheese like cream cheese and camembert/brie – remember to use pasteurised soft cheese for children

STEP 5 **Yoghurt**
Amount - 125mls (4.5 fl oz)

STEP 4 **Cheese**
Amount 15g (1/2 fl oz) (hard cheese e.g. cheddar or parmesan) Once your child tolerates cheese, you can introduce 15g baked cheese on a pizza or baked on other food as well.

STEP 3 **Pancake**
Amount - 1/2 and build up to 1 (see Recipe)

STEP 2 **Muffin**
Amount - 1/2 and build up to 1 (see Recipe)

STEP 1 **Cookie/Biscuit**
Amount - 1 and build up to 3 (see Recipe)

AT EACH OF THE FOLLOWING STEPS
Cookie, muffin, pancake, cheese and yoghurt
It may be advisable in some cases to start with a ¼ or a ½ of that particular food and then over a few days to gradually build up to a whole portion - Please ask your healthcare professional for guidance on this

THE LOWER STEPS ARE DESIGNED TO BE USED WITH HOME MADE RECIPES. THIS IS TO ENSURE THAT EACH STEP HAS THE APPROPRIATE MILK INTAKE. THE RECIPES WILL BE PROVIDED BY YOUR HEALTHCARE PROFESSIONAL
Should you wish to consider locally available store-bought alternatives - seek the advice of your healthcare professional Re: availability

tober 2016

The Imap milk ladder can help you reintroduce milk into your or your child's diet under the supervision of a qualified, regulated health care professional.

Egg ladder

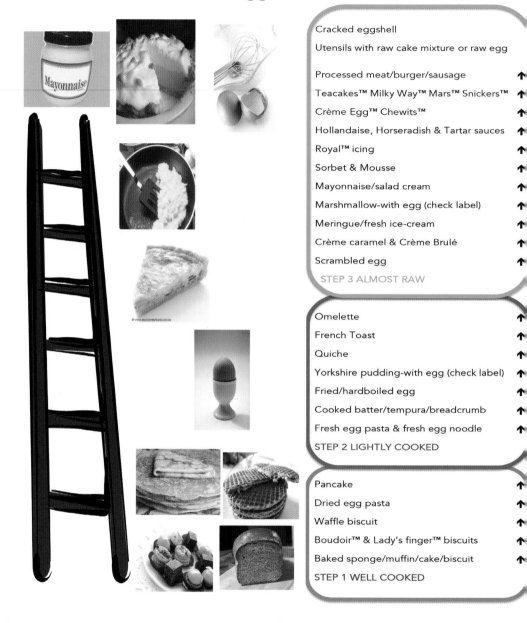

Cracked eggshell

Utensils with raw cake mixture or raw egg

Processed meat/burger/sausage ↑

Teacakes™ Milky Way™ Mars™ Snickers™ ↑

Crème Egg™ Chewits™ ↑

Hollandaise, Horseradish & Tartar sauces ↑

Royal™ icing ↑

Sorbet & Mousse ↑

Mayonnaise/salad cream ↑

Marshmallow-with egg (check label) ↑

Meringue/fresh ice-cream ↑

Crème caramel & Crème Brulé ↑

Scrambled egg ↑

STEP 3 ALMOST RAW

Omelette ↑

French Toast ↑

Quiche ↑

Yorkshire pudding-with egg (check label) ↑

Fried/hardboiled egg ↑

Cooked batter/tempura/breadcrumb ↑

Fresh egg pasta & fresh egg noodle ↑

STEP 2 LIGHTLY COOKED

Pancake ↑

Dried egg pasta ↑

Waffle biscuit ↑

Boudoir™ & Lady's finger™ biscuits ↑

Baked sponge/muffin/cake/biscuit ↑

STEP 1 WELL COOKED

The IFAN egg ladder can help you reintroduce egg into your or your child's diet under the supervision of a qualified, regulated health care professional.

Are you able to predict which children will outgrow their allergies?

Allergies to egg and milk are most likely to be outgrown whilst nuts and fish much less. A number of things can help predict outgrowing such as the size of the allergy test and also the presence of other allergic diseases. Having asthma and eczema are risk factors for allergies not going away. It also depends on which part of the protein you're allergic to. We can do a special allergy test called component testing to help determine this but it's not a definitive answer unfortunately.

Should all children with IgE-mediated food allergies be prescribed adrenaline auto-injectors? And should they avoid 'may contain' labels?

I am not a big believer in blanket prescriptions of adrenaline injectors. It is never a cost factor for me but more about parental anxiety and the social consequences that it brings, if you carry adrenaline when the risk is in fact very low. We need to take an individual approach to risk. We need to carefully risk assess and consider the individual context of each patient. As soon as you get into blanket guidance, bad things can happen as it risks getting in the way of considered judgement. The same applies for the degree of precautions around 'may contains' – it requires individual tailored advice. Everyone's journey is different.

Chapter 10

MANAGING ALLERGIES AT HOME

T he first place you want to make as safe and allergy friendly as possible is your home. This is the place where you can most control your environment and have it set up in the best way for you. It can be stressful living with allergies and make you on high alert, so it is important to have somewhere you can relax.

Shopping with food allergies

When you first shop with food allergies it can be very overwhelming and take ten times longer than usual. It can be daunting to read labels, navigate 'may contains' and check for hidden allergens. The good news is, it does get easier. Although you will still need to check labels every time, as ingredients can change, you will have a better idea of what you are looking for and where to find it.

In the UK, along with the European Union, we have food labelling regulations requiring manufacturers to label the top 14 allergens that most commonly cause reactions. These are:

- milk
- egg
- peanuts
- tree nuts
- cereals containing gluten (including wheat)
- fish
- crustaceans
- molluscs
- soy
- mustard

- sesame
- celery
- lupin
- sulphur dioxide and sulphites

If a food contains these, or any derivatives, then the ingredient must be labelled in bold on any food packaging. This makes it much easier to spot them.

If you are dealing with an allergen outside the top 14, it is a little trickier as you will need to read the ingredients in detail and understand what names different foods may come under. There are also certain things that don't need to be declared in detail if they do not include a top 14 allergen. 'Spices' or 'flavourings' for example may contain multiple ingredients which don't have to be listed individually. If you are unsure, then do not eat it and you can always try to contact the manufacturers for clarification.

'Check everything you eat. You will find allergens hidden in the most bizarre places. Everything that goes in your mouth needs to be checked first.'   *Lauren Gordon*

'May contain' labels

'May contain' labelling is also very confusing. Companies label foods that are at risk of cross contamination during the manufacturing process. This may be because they are made on the same lines as food containing that allergen or because they handle the allergen in the factory. You may come across different types of disclaimers:

- May contain nuts
- Not suitable for milk allergy sufferers
- Made in a factory that also handles egg

Unfortunately, there is no legal guidance on this. Companies do not have to label any products which may have cross contamination issues, they can choose their own wording and some label things when there is very little risk. So it can be difficult to navigate. There is research being done into threshold levels and calls for clearer guidance to make it easier for people living with food allergies.

Manufacturers may distinguish between the risks of cross-contamination from different types of nuts and will label them individually, while many will just use 'nuts' to mean peanuts or tree nuts.

Some foods offer a higher risk of cross-contamination, for example fresh bakery goods, or chocolate, which is sticky and difficult to remove completely from manufacturing equipment. Whether you choose to avoid products with 'may contain' labels or assess contamination risks individually is a personal choice that should be taken based on your tolerance, past reactions, your allergist's advice and what you feel comfortable with. Any food that makes specific free from claims. such as 'milk free' must have followed rigorous controls with no risk of cross contamination. This does not apply to foods labelled 'vegan'.

'Having a child with allergies has taught me a lot about myself, my baby and other people. Thanks to allergies, I can now cook proper, delicious food and I am far more aware of what goes into the food we buy.'
Chloe Wood

Preparing food

There are a number of different ways you may choose to handle preparing food in your own home. Some people choose to create an allergen free home and do not consume anything that their partner or children cannot have. This means that they do not need to worry about any cross contamination and the person with the food allergy can feel relaxed and safe at all times.

Many people won't choose to do this for various reasons. It may be that you have other children with different likes or nutritional needs and you don't want to limit their diet. It may be that you want to continue enjoying the foods you like and help your child understand that other people can eat their allergens around them safely.

If you decide to keep allergens in your house it is important that you have a system in place and take precautionary measures to prevent any mix ups or cross contamination such as:

- Consider only eating allergens once the person with the allergy is in bed or out the house
- Make sure the food is contained on a plate or bowl so no crumbs are left on surfaces
- Wash your hands and mouth after eating them using soap and warm water
- Keep a shelf in your fridge and cupboard for safe foods only
- Wash surfaces and utensils thoroughly with dish soap and warm water
- Use clean knifes and chopping boards every time
- Never double dip e.g. by using a knife in butter and then in the jam jar
- Have a separate toaster or use the grill for allergenic foods

'I grew up in a household that wasn't allergen free and I think this was incredibly beneficial to me. It's not an allergen free world and nor should I expect it to be.' *Nina Modak*

Cosmetics, cleaning products and pet food

In cosmetics or cleaning products, allergens do not need to be labelled in the same way as in food items so it important that you check ingredients carefully. You may also want to be aware of ingredients in pet foods you or children may handle.

If you are allergic to nickel, chemicals or fragrances then this is another area you will need to pay particular attention to. Learn the different names they may fall under, including Latin descriptions and look for natural alternatives to shampoos, soaps and cleaning products. Many people with allergies or eczema will be sensitive to laundry detergents or sun screens and have skin reactions to certain brands.

Medications

If you are allergic to a particular drug you will obviously need to avoid it but also look for where it may be an ingredient in other products – like aspirin in cold remedies. Some medications, supplements and non-prescribed medicines may also be unsuitable for food allergy sufferers as well, due to containing food proteins. Talk to your GP or allergist about these in more detail.

Latex

You may choose not to have latex containing products in your home. Some of these are obvious and easy to avoid, like latex gloves, latex-containing plasters or balloons. Look out for it in other household items too though like rubber bands, babies' dummies, toys, carpet backing, window insulation and some mattresses.

Managing environmental allergies

Environmental allergies can be more difficult to manage than food allergies around the home as they are less easy to see and control. It is almost impossible to banish all levels of dust mites or pollen, so it is a balance of reducing the allergens and managing the symptoms effectively.

Pollen

Pollens can be pervasive and certain pollens are released at different times of year (grass, tree, weed), so it is important to know which ones you react to.

Keep an eye on pollen counts and plan ahead to minimise the impact. Close the doors and windows to limit the amount of pollen inside your home and avoid hanging your washing outside. When you get home, remove your clothing and shower to stop spreading pollen that has stuck to them. A good air purifier with a HEPA filter can also be a sound investment.

When you go outside, use an allergen barrier balm around the outside of your nostrils to try and trap pollen and stop it entering. Wear sunglasses and a brimmed hat to help protect your eyes and you may want to consider wearing a mask if you are walking or cycling for an extended time.

> 'I sleep with the windows closed and have a shower before bed to remove all pollen from my clothes and hair. I use Vaseline at the entrance of my nose to trap the pollen and always go out with large sunglasses on.'
> *Mel Knibb*

Moulds

Mould spores are small and easily released into the air both inside in damp conditions and outside during the autumn. Try and keep your bathroom well ventilated and regularly deep cleaned. Avoid having house plants in your home as moulds can grow in the soil and cause symptoms. Mould likes dark damp corners of a house, so clean regularly behind furniture and in cupboards. It may also be worth getting a mould survey done to identify any potential areas in the home that need treating.

Outside, avoid stirring up compost or leaf piles and don't collect fallen fruit as these can be full of mould spores. You should also be wary of watering the garden, especially after a dry spell, as moulds can be released when the water hits the dry soil.

House dust mites

It is impossible to remove house dust mites completely, but you can help limit them. Beds are a breeding ground as they love warm humid conditions, so buying an anti-allergy mattress cover, duvet and pillowcase can be a good place to start. Wash all your bedding regularly at over 60c and avoid having padded headboards or bedspreads where they can linger. Beds with slats or metal bases are better than divan beds as the air can circulate more. Soft toys are another dust mite trap. Try to minimise the amount your child has, wash these regularly or if they can't be washed, put them in the freezer overnight as the cold will also kill the mites.

Ideally, limit the amount of carpeting in your home and opt for hardwood floors, tiles or laminate instead. Curtains and fabrics can also be an issue. Invest in a good vacuum cleaner with HEPA filters and try to vacuum daily, including under beds, as well as damp dusting surfaces. Central heating and a warm home creates an ideal environment for dust mites so try to turn it down a little when you can.

Pets

Some people are allergic to the dander of animals and others to the saliva and this will make a big difference in how you handle the allergy. You may have allergies to certain animals but still choose to have them in the house, but this will depend on the type and severity of reaction and how much you are able to limit them.

Try and avoid pets licking your hands or skin and wash immediately if they do. Reduce the amount of pet hair around the house by not allowing them in bedrooms and keeping a particular area for them to eat and sleep in. Wash all pet bedding regularly as well as the pets themselves and groom them outside.

Invest in a good vacuum cleaner designed for pet hair and vacuum daily while also limiting the amount of carpet and upholstery in your home which will trap hairs.

Many people are able to continue keeping their pets by following these steps and taking a daily antihistamine. If you are still experiencing symptoms, then the best way to confirm if they are being caused by your pet is to take a holiday away from them and see if symptoms subside. If they do, then you may want to think about re-homing your animal.

'My husband and I have had a cat for 8 years – substantially longer than we've had our sons! We desperately didn't want to have to re-home him so we've taken some practical steps in the house and so far everyone seems OK. I hoover every day, I change my son's clothes every day and his bed every two days, I keep his bedroom door closed to stop the cat going in there and my son knows not to stroke the cat without washing his hands straight afterwards. We've also got hard flooring throughout so cat hair is easy to clean up.'   *Chloe Rowland*

Insect stings

Remember, the likelihood of an insect sting is low in everyday life. Stay calm and try not swat any that land on you. Instead stay still or slowly move away.

Keep foods and drinks covered – never drink out of cans where they can have fallen inside and watch out for sandwiches which they may have crawled into. Try not to walk barefoot outside in case they are in the grass and get someone in to check for nests around your home. Other precautions can include not wearing strong scents or colours that can attract wasps and bees, and avoid picking up fallen fruit.

If you are stung, don't try to pull out the stinger as it can release more venom. Instead, scrape it off with a nail or credit card.

Chapter 11

OUT AND ABOUT WITH ALLERGIES

It is much easier to deal with allergies when you are in your own home as you can control the environment. However daunting it may be to attend social activities, eat out or go on holiday with allergies though, it is important for you and your children to find ways to continue doing everyday activities.

'I have lots of allergies but I don't let them stop me having fun with my friends. My medicines are always with me. I carry them to the playground, or in the car if we go out. The allergies make me who I am. My mummy and daddy say I'm special, but I'm just me. My friends are cool and like to keep me safe which makes me happy!'
Callum Newman (6)

Emergency bag

The first step to heading out and about with allergies is to make sure you are prepared. You should carry any medication with you at all times and it is a good idea to prepare a bag to keep with you or easily grab when you are leaving the house. Things you may want to include:

- Antihistamine
- Adrenaline auto-injectors
- Inhaler and spacer
- Emollient/steroid cream
- Emergency information and care plan
- Wipes to clean hands and surfaces (antibacterial gel does not remove food proteins)
- Safe snacks

You may want to wear an allergy alert bracelet or jewellery in case you are unable to communicate during a reaction, or to remind others about a child's condition. You can also upload emergency and medical information to the home screen of many mobile phones.

Once you have a bag prepared, you should then do some research and a quick risk assessment of where you're going – this will become more instinctive the more you do it. Where are you visiting? What is the activity? Where could your allergens be? What are the risks of a reaction? What can you do to minimise them? What would you do if you had a reaction? This can help you feel more in control and plan the steps you need to take to keep you or your child safe. It will also help you make sure you can be fully included in any activity and minimise any tricky situations.

> 'Be organised! I learnt quickly that I had to be organised and have snacks on hand at every moment in my bag because allergy friendly food was not always available everywhere we went.' *Katharine Spencer*

Whether you are visiting a friend's house, going to the cinema or getting on a train, it is impossible to completely avoid being around all allergens. Try to minimise your exposure, educate those around you and plan ahead. The more prepared you are, the safer you will be and the more confident you will feel in new situations.

Eating out

It can be daunting to put your health in the hands of others, but it is possible to safely eat out with food allergies. All places that serve food have to be able to tell you about any of the top 14 allergens in their meals. Many now have allergen menus at the restaurant or online, although they are not legally obliged to write it down and can deliver the information verbally. Make sure you check these every time as ingredients can change.

The safest way to eat out is to talk to the restaurant beforehand. This will give you a chance to check their attitude to it and also to discuss different options before they are busy with food service. As well as ingredients, you may also want to ask about preparation, what oil food is cooked in and risks of cross contamination. If food is prepared onsite, there is more chance they will be able to adapt dishes. If it is pre-prepared, check they have a full list of ingredients, especially if your allergen falls outside the top 14.

Once you arrive at the restaurant, check with them again and ask to speak to the manager or chef to reiterate your allergies and check they can accommodate you.

It can also be a good idea to carry a chef card with you which lists your allergies and can also include information about cross contamination and your reactions.

When you sit down, use a baby wipe to clean the table or highchair to clear any food residue. When your food arrives, double check with the waiter again as mistakes can be made. If you are ever unsure about something, don't trust the answers you are getting or the staff do not seem to be taking it seriously, then choose not to eat there.

There may be some places that are not safe, or you do not feel comfortable eating at. For example, curry houses or Chinese restaurants may pose a big risk to people with nut or sesame allergies. Or a buffet may cause too many cross contamination concerns. These should all be looked at on an individual basis.

If your friends or family want to eat somewhere you are not comfortable with, then try to talk to them about alternative options. If you still want to go, then ask the restaurant if you can take your own food or substitutes. If not, then you may choose to eat beforehand but still join in socially and enjoy a drink while others eat.

Eating out can be scary, especially if you have had a bad experience before or hear about one. Take small steps, eat at a well-known chain restaurant with an allergen menu or choose something very simple. Ask other people with allergies for recommendations or visit the same place a number of times until you feel more at ease. If you have a bad experience it is important to make the manager aware. If you don't think they are taking it seriously, or need further training, you can report them to the Food Standards Agency. (see: resources)

> 'I use a chef card with all my allergies on and information about cross contamination. It takes away the initial angst of having to explain my multiple food allergies to staff and hoping they will write them down. I still verbally explain but having it written down relieves the pressure for everyone and emphasises the severity of the allergies so there is no confusion. I still like to call ahead to a new restaurant. If they are able to accommodate then they usually appreciate the heads up and if they can't I know I need to find a different restaurant.'   *Allie Bahn*

Travelling

Travelling with allergies can seem like a big step but with a little planning, it can be done as safely as possible.

Before you book a trip, do some research and find out about countries that are safest for your allergen, find recommendations for accommodation or the most allergy friendly airlines.

'We have to remember that food is only one part of the fun of travelling. I have happily travelled to Italy without trying gelato and do not feel like I missed out at all. A new city is so much more than its food and that's where the focus should be; imagine all the new places can you explore. If anything, your wallet will be happy with the hidden benefits of bringing your own food along.'
Kortney Kwong Hing

Flying

There is a lot of fear around flying with allergies, but a few precautions can greatly decrease the likelihood of a serious reaction. If you are allergic to nuts, then you may be able to fly with an airline that makes an announcement and does not serve them while you are onboard or will arrange a buffer zone around you. Take a look at their policies and call ahead to check they are able to do this and tell staff again when you check in and board the plane.

However, you cannot guarantee others have not eaten them before you boarded, or that people will adhere to the announcement. The chances of an airborne reaction are low and it is more likely you will come into contact with your allergen through accidental contact or ingestion. Also, if you suffer from other allergies, then no such accommodations are made so it it is important to do the following:

- Pack any medication, including adrenaline auto-injectors in your hand luggage
- If you are travelling alone, tell an air hostess about your allergies and where your medication is
- Wipe down the tray, armrests and area around you
- Wear long sleeves and trousers, or take a seat cover
- Take your own food
- Choose an early flight, when the plane will be cleaner
- If you are worried about airborne allergies, then consider taking a HEPA mask

If you are allergic to pets, then there is a possibility these may travel on some flights. Contact the airline to talk about the risks and whether they can confirm if your flight will be pet free.

Accommodation

The accommodation you choose will depend on your allergies and what you feel comfortable with. If you are dealing with food allergies, you may want to choose self-catering accommodation so you are able to prepare your own meals. If not, many hotels come with kitchenettes, or at least fridges so you can store your food. Be sure to wash all utensils thoroughly and wipe down surfaces before using them.

If you want to choose catered accommodation, be sure to call ahead before booking and talk to them about your allergies. Are they willing to cater for you? Have they had guests with allergies before? Who will be onsite who understands the risks?

If you are dealing with environmental allergies, especially dust mites or pets, then it is important to make sure wherever you are staying is a safe environment. Many hotels offer hypoallergienic bedding and are willing to do a deep clean of your room if you speak to them in advance. If you want to book self-catering, then ask the provider about whether pets have stayed there in the past and look for somewhere with less carpets and upholstery.

Eating

Eating out with allergies can always be tricky and especially when you are dealing with a foreign language. The most important step is to take an allergy translation card with all your allergies on, which you can use at restaurants or to check ingredients in the supermarket. It is also good to know about labelling laws in the country you are visiting. For example, America only labels for 8 top allergens whereas some other countries don't need to highlight them at all.

If you can, research supermarkets in advance so that you know what is on offer in the place you are visiting. Will you be able to get the dairy-free milk you need? Is there wheat-free bread available? This will help you decide how much you need to take with you.

If you are dealing with a latex allergy you may need to communicate this to staff as latex gloves are still commonly used in food service in some countries.

Medical supplies

Make sure you have adequate supplies of all medications you may need, including lotions, antihistamines or inhalers, as you cannot guarantee you will be able to find more if you run out. Check that they are all in date and are labelled with a doctor's sticker.

You are able to carry your adrenaline auto-injectors in your hand luggage on the plane along with liquids up to 100ml without the need for a doctor's note, although it can be a good idea to carry one anyway. If you need to carry liquids over 100ml, including dairy-free milks, then you are able to do this with a medical exemption letter. You can take as much infant milk in your hand luggage as you need for the journey, although the security staff will probably take it away to be tested.

Auto-injectors can react to extremes of heat, so it is a good idea to keep them in an insulated case and store them in the shade. Think about how you will carry them when you are out and about, on the beach or swimming so you can plan ahead safely.

Emergencies

Nobody wants to have an anaphylactic reaction while abroad, but it is important you have taken steps to know what would happen in an emergency. Make sure you have an up to date care plan with emergency information (translated into the country's language) and multiple auto-injectors.

It is critical that you buy travel insurance and declare all your allergies and medical needs. If you have had a hospital admittance for your allergies in the last few years, some insurers won't cover you, so it is important to shop around. If you have insurance through your bank, or an annual policy, then check with them again before you travel in case any of your treatment or reactions affect your coverage.

It is also a good idea to look up the nearest major hospitals and medical centres for where you are staying, as well as finding the emergency number in the country you are visiting.

Chapter 12

STARTING NURSERY AND SCHOOL

The first time you leave your child in the care of someone else, especially a childcare provider, is always an emotional time but it is particularly daunting when you are dealing with allergies. You will be used to choosing and preparing your child's food, noticing and managing any reactions and keeping them safe each day. The thought of handing this responsibility over to someone else can be very difficult. That is why it is so important to take your time to choose the right childcare, ask lots of questions and build up trust and communication.

Choosing childcare

You need to make sure the any childcare provider fully understands the type and severity of your child's reactions and are willing and able to keep them safe. Start by doing your research, looking at their information online and asking some basic questions about their knowledge and experience of dealing with allergies. It is not essential that they have looked after an allergic child before, but it is important that they take the situation seriously and seem willing to learn.

Next, visit the childcare setting, whether that is a nursery or someone's home and assess the situation. Do they have animals? Where and how is food prepared? What trips do they take? How are meal times managed? Don't be afraid to ask lots of questions. This will give you another chance to see how they react to the challenges. Sit down with them and go through your child's care plan and anything you would expect them to have in place – for example, adrenaline auto-injector training.

It is important that there are strict procedures in place with very young children and that all staff, including those who may work part time or in a support role, are aware of the steps they need to take. They should have a care plan with a picture of your child kept in a prominent place and a well thought out management plan in place.

As well as their safety, it is also important to consider the inclusiveness of the setting. The last thing you want is for your child to be kept safe by being left out of activities. How will they adapt cooking, crafts or outings so that they are safe?

It is important to work with them and help find solutions. Some ideas may be:

- Only feeding your child in a designated highchair with their own plates and cups
- Wiping other children and surfaces before your child gets down
- Choosing park visits with hardstanding rather than grass
- Finding safe alternatives for latex balloons, baking or craft activities

'I was so anxious about sending Elijah to nursery with the severity of his reactions. I didn't know how they would keep him safe. I explained to the nursery management when I visited about Elijah's allergies and they were great. They came out to our home, took a copy of our care plan and created their own risk assessments and protocols for Elijah. They also EpiPen trained every staff member and his picture was up in each room so everyone knew his allergies and what to do around him. This was very reassuring! They also bought him his own high chair, plates, bowls, cups, bottles and cutlery so he wouldn't have reactions and washed and sterilised all of his things separately. They kept him in his high chair until all other children had been cleaned up and the floor was cleaned.'   *Amy Wobbaka*

Allergy management plans

All schools and government run preschools, by law, have to make 'reasonable adjustments' so any child can learn in a safe and adapted environment. (see: resources). Private nurseries and childminders should also work with you to provide a safe environment, but they are not obliged to do so and can refuse to accept your child in their setting. An allergy management plan helps put steps in place to minimise the risk of an allergic reaction and make sure staff know what to do if your child has one.

It's important to start this process once you have found your childcare setting or received your child's school place, so staff have a chance to ask questions, make changes and get everything ready. The first thing to do is to arrange a meeting with the manager or headteacher and class teacher. It is important both these people attend as one will have the most contact with your child but the other is essential for implementing any school wide changes and procedures.

The main goal is to create mutual trust and good communication, so you can take an inclusive and practical approach finding ongoing solutions together.

What a management plan should cover

It is a good idea to set out some clear points you want to cover during the meeting so that everyone has a blueprint of what to expect. Here are some points you may want to include:

- Allergy and adrenaline auto-injector training
- Care plans and management
- Medication storage and access
- Carrying medication during playtime, outdoor or offsite activities
- Schoolwide allergy education
- Classroom snacks, projects, crafts and celebrations
- Physical education, swimming and outdoor play
- Lunchtime seating arrangements, hand washing, cleaning and food management
- Birthdays, parties, school events and cake sales
- School trips

This allows you all to address each point individually, discuss it in depth and know that all the key questions have been covered. You may also need to talk about administering non-emergency medication if your child needs extra emollients for swimming, antihistamines during high pollen counts, or inhalers on a step-down programme after an asthma attack.

Try to work with school as much as possible to create precautions or find solutions. Sometimes allergic conditions can be difficult to understand and many teachers may not have come across them before so it is important to educate the staff in a clear and calm way.

'It can be hard for parents to get through to headteachers and get them to see the value in allergy education. But it's not just about allergies – it's about social development, friendship and looking out for each other. The earlier on you teach them about allergies, the more normal it becomes. Schools also need to focus on inclusion as leaving someone out of an activity to keep them safe can cause a massive wave of emotional disruption. It's very easy to find substitutes and look at different ways to do most things so everyone can participate.'

Hailey Phillips

All staff in your child's school or childcare should be trained to understand the symptoms and how to treat allergic reactions. There are number of ways they can implement this. Most often, the school nurse will be able to run a training session. If not, Anaphylaxis Campaign run workshops and have a comprehensive online training system. (see: resources)

Another essential step is to make sure your child has a clear care plan. The school nurse should contact you to go over this and it is important for you to personalise it for your child's individual symptoms and treatment. You may want to use a care plan your allergy consultant has given you as a guide but also include things such as how your child may describe symptoms, as this can differ to the standard guidance.

The more you can be involved with the whole process from the beginning, the better. This will help build your relationship with the school, make sure everything is in place and hopefully create clear channels of communication. This may include providing a safe snacks list, going along on a school trip or suggesting activities to help children understand allergies – showing them the risks of cross contamination by using glitter is a good one.

Meals

All caterers need to declare the top 14 allergens and also take steps to provide your child with a safe school meal. Talk directly to the kitchen staff if meals are prepared onsite, or to the caterers if they are brought in. They should be able to suggest substitutions, discuss ingredients and take the time to plan a safe menu. Be sure any extra staff – like dinner ladies, support staff or servers – are aware of your child's allergies and do not risk any cross contamination. You may feel more comfortable, at least initially, with your child taking a packed lunch. Talk to staff about seating arrangements, handwashing, cleaning and working with the children to stop food sharing.

Food bans

Many settings are now 'nut free' and this can be very reassuring for parents who are dealing with nut allergies. However, these bans are very difficult to police and there is no evidence that banning an allergen reduces incidents. They can also be discriminatory for families dealing with multiple allergies, who will find it is much harder to ban all the foods their child is allergic to. It is unlikely that a nursery or school would agree to ban all dairy, for example.

Food bans should not be a replacement for staff and children having allergy training and clear care plans in place. The European Academy of Allergy and Clinical Immunology, along with Allergy UK, do not advise blanket banning of allergens. Instead, they encourage parents and schools to devise a good management plan together. This may include the control of allergens – for example, keeping classrooms allergen free or not allowing snacks in the playground.

Facing challenges

Many childcare providers and schools will be very willing and keen to make sure your child is as safe as possible. However, sometimes you may face resistance, especially if you are dealing with a non-IgE food allergy or non-life-threatening conditions like hay fever. Many people struggle to understand these conditions and the adverse effects they can have on quality of life and your child's ability to learn.

If you are facing challenges or feel that the allergy management plan is not being put in place satisfactorily, then talk to the headteacher. If they are still resistant, approach the Special Educational Needs (SEN) co-ordinator or school nurse who should be able to support you. To take the matter further, contact the school's governors, your local council or talk to Allergy UK. Every school needs to make reasonable adjustments to allow your child to learn in a safe environment. There are two pieces of legislation that can support you in getting an appropriate management plan in place: 'Supporting pupils at school with medical conditions' and the Disability Discrimination Act, which covers severe allergies. (see: resources)

Teaching children about their allergies

As well as working closely with the school, it is important your child understands their allergies and can help protect themselves. It is natural to want to shield and protect you child but it is essential that you help them understand and manage them.

'Always check with an adult about the food, bring your own food to places you are going if you aren't sure what food will be there and only let a trusted adult or you touch your food. Tell people what you're allergic to and explain what happens if you eat that food. Make sure people who are going to be around you know what you look like when you are having an allergic reaction because you might not be able to speak. Living with food allergies is okay. It might take some time to get used to. I don't remember life before food allergies. So for me it's not that bad.'

Freya Spencer (12)

The earlier you can start talking to them the better, as this will help them see their allergies as a normal part of life and not something to be anxious about. While it obviously needs to be taken seriously, it is important not to project any of your fear or anxieties on to them.

Even young children can start learning about their allergies. Use explanations and language they can understand. So you may say they can't have a certain food because it would make them poorly or make their tummy hurt. Or explain how their body might react if they come into contact with an environmental allergen. As they get older, you can talk about symptoms in a bit more detail so they know what to look out for.

Make it a part of everyday conversation. So if you are dealing with food allergies, involve them in shopping, cooking or eating out and explain why you are choosing something or making something in a certain way. As they get older, you can help them read labels or even support them to order their own food. It is also important to explain what their allergens look like and where they might hide. Many children have no idea what a nut actually looks like! Make sure they understand that they must never share food or eat anything that has not been given to them by a trusted adult.

Sometimes allergens are less tangible – like pollens, dust mites or bee stings. Talk about these with them, explain any precautions you take and why you may choose to things in a certain way. Help them to manage their allergies by looking at the pollen count, damp dusting surfaces or taking their medication with them.

For young children, role play and stories can work really well as it helps them to process different situations. Get a toy kitchen, including some of their allergens like milk or egg, and when they are making meals explain what they can't have or how they could make it instead. There are some really good books out there as well. Those written by children themselves can be especially good, as they are written in a language and way they can connect with.

'Explain your child's allergy to them in an age appropriate way. Be sure to talk to them as honestly as possible without scaring them and teach them the importance of checking what's in their food, not accepting food if they don't know what's in it and having their inhaler or EpiPen with them at all times. They will learn from you, so stay as calm as possible if they are having a reaction. Teach them how to explain their allergies to others and how to say no and how to ask for help if they need it.'   *Laura Kenny*

As children get older, they can take more responsibility for their allergies. Once they go to school, they need to be able explain to others what they need to avoid and understand when they have to say no to any food or activity that is offered. It is also essential that they know what a reaction may feel like, when to tell an adult and what the treatment will be.

If they have been prescribed an adrenaline auto-injector, then use a practice one to show them how it is used. Try to minimise any fear by explaining exactly what it does, letting them have a go with a practice pen which does not have a needle and helping them understand when and why you may need to use it.

An adult caregiver will need to be trained to use the auto-injector and keep hold of them for younger children. As they get older though, and definitely by the time they go to high school, they will need to feel confident in carrying and administering their own. Some simple steps to help them take control of their own allergies are:

- Teach them to always wash their hands before eating
- Help them wipe down surfaces
- Read ingredients with them
- Choose a medication bag and allow them to pack it
- Show them how to use their medication and let them administer it, if they can
- Make sure they check they have it each time they leave the house
- Use role play to practice declining foods or activities

While your child needs to know these things, they cannot be expected to fully understand and not make mistakes at such a young age. This is why it is so important that the teachers and people caring for them are able to take steps to minimise the risk and know what to do in an emergency.

'It's hard not always being able to eat things your friends can, especially at lunchtimes at school but when we do get safe foods we don't have to share with anyone! Always remember you are not the only one who has allergies – there are other people who have them too!'   *Millie Peacock (8)*

Birthday parties

Once your child hits school age, they will probably start getting invited to numerous birthday parties as well as other play dates. These can be anxiety inducing for allergy parents but avoiding them is not a long-term solution and is not good for you or your children.

Taking some simple steps can help you feel more confident in approaching them:

- **Talk to the host when you get the invitation** so there is enough time to address any concerns like menus or balloons
- **Call the venue** if it is being held externally and liaise with them directly
- **Get your child's plate of food first** at buffets, before any cross contamination from sticky fingers and ask parents to keep labels so you can check ingredients
- **Take your own food** if you are unsure or want to make it easier for the host. Remember to think about birthday cake and treats for the party bags
- **Stay and supervise** if your child is young or if you are concerned

'For parties and events, the easiest thing is to bring your own allergy safe food. Ask the host beforehand what type of party food will be served. Then you can match your party lunchbox with similar food to what will be served, so your child won't feel left out. If it's family or a close friend you can offer to help, then you can check packaging and see what is safe to eat. It is a nice idea to bring some allergen free food to share also as then there is something everyone can have.'
Laura Kenny

Expert Insight: Managing allergies in childhood

Amena Warner
Head of clinical services
Allergy UK

What do parents need to look for when choosing a childcare provider?

When parents are choosing childcare they need to ask lots of questions and find out what their knowledge base is and what they know about managing allergies. Ask if they have or had other children with allergy, particularly if there is a risk of serious reactions, do they know how to deal with these, have they had training? Parents need to be proactive and work in partnership with childcare providers. As long as they are receptive, you can put a management plan in place together, with a picture of the child, what they are allergic to, what medication they have been prescribed and what symptoms to look out for. It is a bit like fire training – people need to know where the fire extinguishers are, as well as how to put out a fire and when to get help. These are usually in policies and procedures, so you need to make sure the childcare provider has these to look at how children with allergy are looked after safely.

What do you think about nut bans in schools?

I completely understand why parents would want to avoid something that could harm their child and how precious their child's life is. But it's a very unrealistic environment. Research shows those who are in schools with nut bans have more reactions. It is more important for children, schools and friends to all be allergy aware. The child needs to be able to live as normal a life as they can. There is lots of scaremongering out there. That fear is projected on to that child, rather than talking sensibly about how to keep them safe. It is about how we responsibly manage all allergies.

How can parents help young children manage their allergies?

Bring it down to their level of understanding. Read them stories, role play, show them what different foods look like. It has to become the norm. You don't want to frighten them so they become obsessed with it but they need to understand it's there in the background. They should have some knowledge – what a reaction feels like and to tell an adult. Try to teach them to advocate for themselves from a young age so it doesn't become a barrier and they think they can't tell anyone. Allergy management plans should include what they might say or how they would describe a reaction, as it can be different to the medical explanation.

> 'I have allergies and asthma and sometimes it's a bit scary but I play, go on holiday and make the best chocolate cake with no eggs. Just always carry your medicine and tell someone if you feel unwell. Don't worry, your allergies don't need to stop you having lots of fun with your friends.'
> *James Amoscato (5)*

Chapter 13

YOUNG PEOPLE AND TEENAGERS

As children get older, it is important to help them take responsibility for their allergies and learn to manage them. Once a child is in high school they should be supported to carry their medication and know how to administer an adrenaline auto-injector if they need one.

The most high-risk age group for a fatal allergic reaction is 16-24 as they are naturally more risk taking. If they have not had a serious allergic reaction since they were young, then the concept can seem very abstract and they may just think their parents are overreacting. This is why it is important to help them understand their allergies.

'The start of secondary school was a turning point, as it was when my son started to carry his own EpiPens. He also practised using a trainer pen and we taught his friends how to give the EpiPen in case of a reaction. We've encouraged him to self-advocate. He speaks up at school if he's concerned and outside of school we've shown him how to read labels for his allergens and encouraged his interest in cooking. When we eat out, he now orders his own food and explains his allergies. The next challenge will be increased independence and eating out with friends on his own.'

Sarah Smith

If they have food allergies, help them read food labels, do the shopping and cook for themselves so that they understand what goes into their food and how to prepare safe meals. Let them order a meal in a restaurant and communicate their allergies and needs to others.

If they are dealing with asthma or environmental allergies, help them risk assess a situation and talk through different ways they could manage it. Encourage them to take their own precautions and manage their medication.

'When you are a teenage boy, your allergies are literally one of the last things on your hierarchy of important things (hovering around homework). Your underdeveloped brain is constantly pulling you between sports, girls, music, clothes, being cool etc. The desire to fit in is one of the biggest threats for staying safe with allergies as it can often lead to risk-taking behaviour. It can be the reason why a teen purposely leaves their epinephrine at home or why they stop telling new friends about their allergies out of fear that they will be judged. Teenage boys will try to shake their parents off trying to convince them that they have their allergies under control. But during these years, it's so important for parents to keep the conversation going and keep tabs on how their teen as they start to take on more responsibility for their own health condition.' *Kyle Dine*

Many allergy clinics will recommend that children get retested around this time and even undertake a challenge in hospital. This may seem daunting or even unnecessary, but it is a good way to help young people address their allergies. If the tests come back negative or they pass a challenge, then it means they do not need to avoid things any longer and take away any unnecessary restrictions or anxiety. If the tests are positive or they fail a challenge, then it reinforces the need to take their allergies seriously. The more they understand their allergies, can advocate for themselves and know what to do in an emergency, the more empowered they will feel. This can help reduce anxiety, make them more likely to carry their medication and make sure allergies do not hold them back.

'I manage my allergies by making my own packed lunch with safe food I can eat, ensuring I have my EpiPens and emergency action plan in my school bag at all times, and using my inhaler before exercise. I also regularly talk about how to manage my allergies with my parents. My tips for other teenagers would be always carry two EpiPens and don't be afraid to speak up in front of your teachers and friends if anything makes you feel unsafe.' *Simon Marks (15)*

School and social activities

Starting high school can present new challenges. Your child will probably need to carry their own medication and be able to advocate for themselves more independently. It is still important you work closely with the school to create a safe and inclusive environment. Some areas you may need to discuss are:

- Staff allergy awareness and training
- Allergy awareness education for pupils
- Medication storage and access during physical activity
- Cookery classes
- Catering
- School trips and residentials
- After school clubs

Teenagers and young people will want to have more freedom to meet up with their friends and spend time without you. It can be difficult to let go as an allergy parent, but it is important they are able to do this, while still managing their allergies responsibly.

Try to involve them in speaking up about their allergies, risk assessing a situation and putting steps in place to manage it. This may involve talking to the person who runs an organised club or a parent at whose house they will be staying, or showing their friends how to use an adrenaline auto-injector.

If your child is going out without adult supervision, then role play different situations, discuss how they would handle them and make sure they are fully prepared. Most importantly, they must always carry their auto-injector if they are at risk of anaphylaxis. You may also want to:

- Buy them some allergy alert jewellery
- Upload an emergency app on their phone
- Find a medication bag they feel confident carrying
- Research allergy friendly brands and places to eat
- Talk about how to handle parties, kissing and alcohol with allergies

Stigma/bullying

It is important that young people are not embarrassed about talking about their allergies and can educate their friends about their condition. Encourage them to tell friends about their allergies and explain what they need to do to manage them or how to help in an emergency. Usually friends are very understanding, look out for each and an important support network for young people. Reading about, or talking to, other young people with allergies can also be helpful. Look for blogs, social media or support groups to help connect with others who understand. Help your child realise that anyone who teases them or doesn't take it seriously is not someone they want in their life.

This openness will help keep them safe, make them less likely to take risky decisions but also lower the likelihood of bullying. Unfortunately, bullies are always looking for something different in people to pick on and when allergies aren't taken seriously this can have emotional and physical consequences.

If you think your child is being bullied, talk to the school and encourage them to help educate the other children about the consequences of allergies. Make sure they take any incidents seriously, and if your child's life has been threatened or put in danger, contact the police.

'Bullies in general have a bad rap. We are quick to paint them as a bad kid, but no one is born a bully. It comes from someone, something, somewhere. Food allergy bullying seems incomprehensible for those directly affected by allergies. But they most likely have limited experience with food allergy or were given misinformation. Unfortunately, I've come across kids who ask questions such as "are you faking your allergies?" which makes me believe this attitude is also being learned at home through adults who haven't been properly educated either. It's up to our schools, parents and communities to teach kids about food allergies early in life. It's important to include messaging not only on the condition itself, but to emphasize empathy for those dealing with allergies. In my experience, when kids are given the chance to learn about allergies in an age-appropriate fashion, they take it!'
Kyle Dine

Leaving home

When your child leaves home, it is a difficult time for any parent and it is natural for everyone to feel apprehensive. The young person is excited about the new stage of their life but also nervous about coping on their own, while the parent is sad to see them go and worried about them staying safe.

Like anything concerning allergies, the more planning and preparation you do, the smoother things will go. The years leading up to a young person leaving home are really important as it gives them a chance to take responsibility for their allergies in a safe and supportive environment. Parents can slowly hand over different tasks, from shopping and cooking to managing medication and keeping an allergy safe home.

Accommodation

Whether someone is going to university, or just moving out of home, accommodation will be a major consideration. Where is most suitable? Who will you live with? How will you keep it allergy safe?

It is important that anyone you are living with is aware of your allergies. Discuss what they can do to limit your exposure and what to do if you have a reaction. The fewer people who you share with, the easier this will be to manage. If you are going to university, then you may want to ask for smaller, self-catering accommodation so you can manage your needs effectively. For food allergies, You may want to:

- Take separate chopping boards and utensils
- Keep your own cupboard or shelves for your food
- Explain to people how to eat your allergens safely

If you are dealing with environmental allergies, then you will need to consider your surroundings. Think about:

- Where the accommodation is and any trees, mould or damp that could trigger your symptoms
- Flooring, upholstery and how you will keep the place clean
- Do people have pets or have they had them in the home previously?

'The thing that makes the biggest impact in feeling comfortable with allergies at uni is that my friends are all aware of it. Most importantly, the people I live with all have the knowledge of the severity of it. Socialising can be tricky sometimes since lots of it involves food but since all my friends know about my allergies, they usually make sure I feel comfortable anywhere we go. I usually go to places that have allergy menus but are also cost effective. Being at uni with allergy was originally slightly worrying but i have found many people who have intolerance and allergies so that makes it easier. I feel like it doesn't hinder my university experience.' *Emily Chapman*

Expert Insight: Managing allergies for young people

Grace Brocklehurst
Anaphylaxis Campaign

Why are young people at a high risk of having an anaphylactic reaction?

Many young people may never have had a reaction, or only as a young child, so they don't understand why they need to carry adrenaline auto-injectors and think their parents are being overprotective. We got lots of parents calling around the time children transition to the adult service at 16 or when they are going to university or travelling. Parents need to slowly hand over responsibility – let them do the food shop, cook and order in restaurants while you are right beside them. Then you can empower them.

How can their peers be educated?

In schools it is important that not just staff but the whole school understand allergies. Awareness days and assemblies help. It can be helpful for teenagers to see hard-hitting videos like Anaphylaxis Campaign's 'Take the kit' to help them understand the severity of a reaction. Bullying in any form is not acceptable, but for pupils with severe allergies the potential consequences are deadly. Allergy bullying is sadly still seen and should be treated seriously like any other bullying. If parents think the school is not taking it seriously, then take it to the headteacher, governors or local council.

What tips do you have for people leaving home or going away to university?

It's good to inform university and ask for a smaller flat so it is easier to manage. Young people should explain to their flatmates about their allergies, learn to make basic meals and keep their food and utensils separate. It is important to pre-plan for everything, know you have your medication, where to get safe food and that the people you are with know about your allergies.

What do people need to think about when socialising?

Alcoholic drinks can contain allergens. Risk assess a situation – if there's a cocktail, stick to wine. If there are peanuts, move away. Go out with people you feel comfortable with and tell them. Carrying adrenaline auto-injectors can be tricky on a night out. We hear through our helpline boys especially find this hard due to not having a handbag, but it is essential to take it. Carry a doctor's note in case security question it and if they won't let you in with it, you need to leave. Also, always make sure you have safe snacks for the end of the evening.

Chapter 14

ALLERGIES IN ADULTS

A lot of focus is often on managing allergies in children, especially with the rise of childhood allergies. However, managing allergies as an adult presents its own set of challenges. You may have been dealing with your whole life, or it may be something you have suddenly had to get used to. Either way, it is important to take active steps to protect yourself while continuing to lead a full life.

Adult onset allergies

It is possible to develop allergies at any age, even without a history of them previously and up to 15 per cent of allergies start in adulthood. They often develop after an illness or hormonal change, which may disrupt the immune system or your gut health and affect the way the body views previously safe substances.

It can be a big shock to suddenly face life with allergies when they haven't been a concern before, or to have to deal with new or more severe symptoms. They may be affecting your daily quality of life or causing you anxiety.

The first step is to do your research, talk to a qualified allergist and make sure you really understand what you are dealing with, what to avoid and how to manage any reactions. Then it is a good idea to find some support. There are lots of online groups, or Anaphylaxis Campaign runs in-person meet ups.

In the workplace

Many people feel awkward about addressing their allergies at work and worry about it affecting their job or career.

It is not necessary to mention your allergies when you apply for a job, although you may choose to. It is a good idea to talk about them once you accept any offer though. This gives your employer a chance to put provisions in place, discuss it with HR and work with you to set anything up.

The Disability Discrimination Act means people with allergies have a right to fair and reasonable treatment at work and employers cannot discriminate against you in:

- Recruitment and Selection
- Contractual Terms
- Promotion
- Training
- Dismissal

They must be willing to make reasonable adjustments for you to work in a safe environment, which may include providing alternative equipment or duties. If you feel you are not being treated fairly, talk to HR, approach your trade union if you have one, or talk to Citizens Advice.

Many people want to avoid appearing awkward or standing out so they don't discuss their allergies at work. However, it is important at least a few key people know if you are at risk of a serious reaction, so they can act quickly if you go into anaphylaxis.

> 'It's hard because everything from simple tea making, team events, socials and seminars includes food. My desk drawer is full of safe snacks. I nearly always make the drinks myself as things are just so instinctive, like stirring a mug of tea with the same spoon that's been in a milky one. On the whole it's getting easier every year though as restaurants get better at catering and supermarkets provide more and more safe food.'
> *Ruth Holroyd*

Allergies and the military

Employers cannot discriminate against you because of your allergies but unfortunately, there may be times when your allergies limit or prevent you from taking the career choice you wish. One of these is following a career in the armed services. It is important that all serving military personnel are fit and do not have any conditions that could put themselves or others at risk. While most people with allergies are fit and well between reactions, if someone suffers one on deployment it could be difficult to handle.

If you have a severe food allergy and need to carry an adrenaline auto-injector then you are unable to serve in the armed forces as they cannot guarantee you will always have access to safe food. They are exempt from the Disability Discrimination Act which is why they are able to make this rule. In cases where you have not had a severe reaction for a long time or were diagnosed in childhood, then you may be able to get further tests and assessments to see if you are still at risk.

It is important to be honest about your medical history as any mention of allergies will be flagged up in your GP records. Asthma and eczema may also be a concern, but these would be addressed on a more individual basis to see if they pose a problem to active service.

Occupational allergies

Employers have a responsibility to manage health and safety at work and assess the risks of any harmful substances or the possibility of people developing occupational allergies. It is difficult to know how sensitive an individual will be to a substance though and often, once the symptoms and trigger have been recognised, it is too late to prevent the allergy continuing.

In cases where an allergy may prevent you doing your job, or if you have developed an occupational allergy through being exposed to something at work, you may be eligible for immunotherapy. Pollen, pet or venom allergies can be desensitised through a series of injections or capsules taken at home over an extended period to limit the reactions. (see more: chapter 7)

Pubs, clubs and concerts

Drinking, clubbing and concerts can be tricky to manage with food allergies. If you have an allergy to alcohol, then obviously you will avoid it, but you also need to be careful with other allergies. Many drinks contain sulphites and you can also find milk in wine. Be careful with any cocktails or liqueurs and it is generally safer to stick to simple drinks unless you are sure of the ingredients.

Drinking alcohol can also impair your judgement and your ability to deal with an allergic reaction. So be sensible and make sure the people you are socialising with are aware of your allergies and know where your medication is.

> 'It's important that at least a few people around you know about your allergies. Make them aware of exactly what your allergens are, what happens during a reaction, where your medication and information is and more importantly, how or when to use it.'   *Midge Peacock*

Some bars and pubs still serve loose nuts so plan how you would manage this situation. If you are allergic to latex you will need to watch out for balloons or stick to open air venues if you are dealing with fragrance allergies. If you feel too uncomfortable, then you may want to leave or just move to a different area.

If you carry adrenaline auto-injectors then it is important to have them with you at all times, even on a night out. This can be easier for women who will generally carry a handbag but trickier for men. Some people have had issues with security staff wanting to take their adrenaline auto-injectors away. Ideally, if you know where you are going in advance, call them up and explain your medical needs or carry a doctor's note with you. If they are still resistant, ask to speak to management and ultimately, if they won't comply, it is not worth the risk. Leaving your auto-injectors in their office or other location is simply not a safe option.

Think about snacks and drinks for when you head home as well. Your friends may want to get a curry or a kebab, so it is a good idea to have some safe options ready for yourself.

Dating and relationships

The last thing you want to do is talk about kissing on a first date but when you're dealing with allergies it might be necessary! When you are trying to impress a potential partner, it is natural not to want to make things awkward or raise any difficulties, but it is important to stay safe. Plus, if they don't take the conversation well, you will soon know if they are not the one for you.

When you are getting physically intimate with someone, the last thing you want is to have an allergic reaction so think ahead. If you have food allergies, you will need to talk to them about avoiding eating your allergens when you are going to see them and making sure they have cleaned their teeth before any kissing takes place. If you are allergic to perfumes or pets, then make sure you have this conversation so they do not have anything on them that could trigger a reaction. If you are allergic to latex, it is important to be prepared with latex free condoms and take responsibility for having safe sex.

'The good thing about having food allergies and dating is that you have to be open, upfront, and any awkwardness goes away quite fast. Let's face it, if you don't talk about kissing from the get-go, it may never happen. Plus you get to wean out the baddies pretty quickly. Seeing how someone reacts to your food allergies is a telling sign of whether they are someone you want to be with. If they don't want to list off what they ate before a kiss, are they worth dating? Openness will become a foundation to your relationship, and that can only be a good thing!' *Kortney Kwong Hing*

Pregnancy

It is natural when you consider having children of your own to worry about how your allergies will affect them. Will you pass them on? Is there anything you can do to prevent them? How will you handle your own allergies around them?

The advice during pregnancy is to continue to eat a balanced and healthy diet, only avoiding any foods that you are allergic to. If you do not have food allergies, then you should include all regular allergens in your diet. You will probably be able to continue taking most medication you are on but talk to your doctor about it in more detail. If you have a severe allergic reaction while you are pregnant then you should use your adrenaline auto-injector as normal as risks to your unborn baby are minimal.

Allergies do have a genetic link and around half of children born to atopic parents will also develop them in some form. There is some emerging evidence that taking a probiotic and fish oil during your third trimester may help improve your gut health and prevent your child developing allergies. (see more: chapter 17)

Parenting

The good news is, having allergies yourself means you are in a stronger position to spot the symptoms and understand the causes if your child has them. Always mention your own medical history when talking to doctors about your child's suspected allergies.

Recent studies show that it is important to introduce allergenic foods early to children at high risk of developing allergies. (see more: chapter 17). If you have allergies yourself, it can be difficult to know how to do this safely. Talk to your doctor about the risks and how to approach this. It may be something your partner can manage, or you can put precautions in place like wearing gloves, or only letting your child only eat in their highchair and thoroughly cleaning the area afterwards.

Another thing you may want to think about is helping your child understand your allergies. Children are very open and receptive, but it is important to explain anything they may be concerned about. Talk to them about your symptoms, why you can't have pets or certain foods and how you treat any reaction. They are likely to have many questions as they grow up and try to address them in an age appropriate way, managing any fears and anxieties they may have.

'Having allergies forces you to practice being the type of person everyone wants to be. To be honest, confident, stand up for what you believe in. I believe it instils a sense of responsibility and conscientiousness for others. At least I believe we can cultivate these qualities by using our allergies as a tool to make us better human beings.'   *Nina Modak*

Expert Insight: Allergies in adults

Dr Stephen Till
Consultant in adult allergy

What circumstances bring people to your adult allergy clinic?

We see some people with adult onset allergies, also some who have had allergies as children but fallen off the radar and then others transitioned from the paediatric service for continuing care. The latter group may have been followed up for years and in many cases we need to try and transition them to be more independent.

What are the main problems you see with allergy diagnosis in adults?

People attribute to food many symptoms are caused elsewhere by other things so it is important to identify what is a true allergy. There are lots of practitioners out there who are not trained in allergy and providing dubious or wrong advice. There is no other speciality I can think if where that is so widespread or accepted by the public. I think it is partly because real allergy clinics are thin on the ground and overwhelmed. For example, it is common for someone to go the GP because they have been getting an itchy mouth when they eat nuts. A blood test may be performed and they may then be told that they are allergic to nuts and to totally avoid them. But this is often only a minor issue caused by birch pollen allergy (oral allergy syndrome) which needs to managed differently and strictly avoiding all nuts is generally unnecessary. So, access to allergy experts who can run the right tests and interpret them properly is vital. Also, people rely on tests performed by alternative practitioners that have virtually no value. In many cases this is because they are not allergic but strongly believe that foods trigger their symptoms, so in desperation they seek answers elsewhere.

What are the most common adult onset allergies?

Statistically, the most common adult onset allergy is oral allergy syndrome to fresh fruits or tree nuts. The most common adult onset anaphylactic allergy is crustaceans, probably as because people are exposing themselves to new varieties they may not have eaten before. Adult onset allergy has been highlighted as a priority area of research by the Food Standards Agency.

What problems do you see for adults managing their allergies?

People can feel very oppressed by their allergies as adults. It can all be very stressful having to constantly declare your medical history for example when at work/college/school, out socialising, or eating out with colleagues or clients. Occasionally we hear issues in the workplace with colleagues not taking severe allergies seriously and even making jokes, which is a form of bullying. There are sometimes issues with hotdesking where people are expected to work at different desks, not knowing what someone has been eating there beforehand. For those with severe allergies this can be a difficult experience. Foreign travel can be a problem too, as in some cultures food allergies are much rarer. Quality of life is the number one issue we need to address but there is virtually no adult psychological support available in my experience. Some adults also suffer greatly after experiencing a bad reaction.

Is there any oral immunotherapy available for adults?

We are starting the first study into peanut immunotherapy in adults at Guy's Hospital in the near future.

Chapter 15

SUPPORT AND PSYCHOLOGICAL EFFECTS

One thing that can often feel overlooked when you are dealing with allergies is the psychological impact it can have. There is a lack of support services out there, but it is an area that more allergy clinics are recognising and trying to find ways to address.

Often, because allergies are hidden and reactions aren't happening daily, it can seem to others like it is all under control. However, when you are facing the challenge of keeping yourself or a child safe, the anxiety can become overwhelming. Or if your symptoms are affecting your daily life, this can also affect your mental health. This can be heightened if you are new to dealing with allergies, after a reaction or when you are faced with a situation you are unfamiliar with.

The first thing to remember is that you are not alone. Up to 20 per cent of people dealing with allergies struggle daily with the fear of a possible asthma attack or anaphylactic shock.[1]

Guilt

Many people feel guilty when dealing with allergies. This may because you feel you are being a burden on others or because you feel responsible for your child developing them. This is also exacerbated after a reaction if you feel it was your fault or could have done something to prevent it.

Self-doubt and denial

As a parent you may second guess your child's symptoms, especially if you are not getting the right support elsewhere. You may also react by downplaying things, convincing yourself a reaction is not happening. This can be particularly dangerous during anaphylaxis.

Exhaustion

Dealing with allergies can be physically and emotionally exhausting. The symptoms can leave you drained and so can managing or preventing them. If you are looking after a child, you may be missing sleep to care for them which makes everything else so much harder.

Helplessness

It is normal to feel that living with allergies is not fair and to have a certain level of anger or frustration about your situation. You may feel helpless or out of control, especially if you are experiencing regular symptoms or reactions.

Fear and anxiety

Many people feel fear and anxiety about their allergies, wondering when or how they will react and feeling out of control. Parents can feel particularly anxious about keeping their children safe. This can become overwhelming, especially after a serious reaction, and it is important to find ways to cope with your feelings.

> 'The anxiety of having a child with severe food allergies never goes away but you learn to cope. Research support groups for your child's condition and talk to parents who have been through or are going through the same thing. It's good to know you are not going through this journey alone. You will also find parents who have made it out the other side. Their stories are good for you to know, to give you comfort on your darkest days.'
>
> *Katharine Spencer*

Relationship issues

Allergies can affect your relationships with your partner, your family and your friends. They may lead to arguments at home, especially if you feel your partner is not taking things seriously. It can also be difficult for others to understand and you may feel unsupported by family members, or stop going out and socialising, which can impact friendships.

Loneliness and isolation

You may start limiting your social interaction if you feel people don't understand, you are anxious about your allergies, or if the symptoms are becoming difficult to manage. This can lead to loneliness and isolation. It is essential to build a support network to help combat this, whether in person or online.

Helping children with allergies

Allergies can also have a psychological impact on children coping with them. They may feel scared, upset or anxious. They may also feel self-conscious, worried about being different or how their friends may treat them. It is essential to talk openly with them to address their feelings and build coping strategies together. Finding support groups, books or online communities where they can talk to other children their own age with allergies can also help.

If they are scared of tests or challenges, have food anxiety, are struggling after a reaction or their worry is affecting their daily life, then talk to your doctor about how a play specialist or psychologist may be able to help.

'Allergies affect children more emotionally than physically as they get older. We need to give them the right information and help them to have a positive mindset – Look what I *can* do and what we *can* eat.'
Hailey Phillips

Impact on other children

Other children in the family can also be affected. Children without allergies may feel left out, as though their sibling is getting more attention. They may also feel scared or worried themselves about how to keep them safe. Try to involve them as much as possible, talk to them about their worries and spend time alone with them so they get individual attention as well.

'When my sister was little, I was really cautious. I was always telling people what her allergies were to make sure they didn't give her food. I wanted her to be safe.'
JP Knibb (9)

How to cope

Allergies, the chronic disruption they can cause and the possibility of a serious reaction are a difficult thing to live with every day. It is easy for fears and worries to consume your thoughts and stop you leading a normal life. Some steps you can take are:

- **Understand your allergies fully.** Knowledge is power so talk to your allergist, do some research and understand as much as you can about your allergies, what reactions they could cause and how you can manage them.
- **Have an emergency plan.** Part of taking control of your allergies is knowing exactly what you would do in an emergency. Carry a written plan, discuss it with your allergist and share it with friends and family.

- **Carry your medication at all times and know how to use it.** Many people are scared of using an auto-injector when in fact, it is very easy with barely any adverse effects. Use a practice pen so you feel prepared in an emergency.
- **Build your confidence** by taking small steps to visit a new place, eat out or talk to someone about your allergies.
- **Find a support network.** Talking to other people who are also dealing with allergies will help you feel less alone. There are many online support groups, or Anaphylaxis Campaign also run in person ones too.
- **Pass on your knowledge.** Helping others who are at the beginning of their allergy journey, or who are also struggling, can help you find a positive angle to your experiences.
- **Limit your information intake.** Understanding your allergies is empowering but reading too much can have the opposite effect. Spending a long time in online forums or reading about fatal reactions may distort your view of how likely a severe reaction may be.
- **Seek help.** If the anxiety is becoming overwhelming, or you are struggling to cope after a severe reaction, talk to your GP or find a trained therapist who can offer further support.

'I make sure I've researched as much into things as possible so I've got all the information and can then tell myself I've made my decisions based on all the relevant facts.'
Chloe Rowland

In extreme cases, anxiety can develop into panic attacks, with symptoms mimicking that of an allergic reaction. You may be struggling more than you realise and need to seek further support from your GP or a trained psychologist or councillor if you:

- Avoid social activities because of your allergies
- Have trouble sleeping due to worry
- Show physical signs of anxiety – sweating, shaking, rapid breathing
- Find it difficult to stop thinking about allergies
- Have intrusive negative thoughts

Expert Insight: Psychological impact of allergies

Rebecca Knibb
Chartered Psychologist, Associate Professor in Psychology and Health Psychology Practitioner

Why do allergies have a psychological impact on people?

Allergies are a very unusual long-term condition. It's hidden, you often aren't unwell and don't have reactions every day. You can't see it; it's not tangible and those allergens hide. Allergies are so unpredictable. The risk of dying is very small but that doesn't reduce anxiety because you still think it could be me or my child.

How can parents help themselves to manage the anxiety?

The biggest thing parents face is that fear and worry. There are certain trigger points – initial diagnosis, children starting nursery, school trips or the routine changes. Then when children become teenagers and want to go out on their own you have to readjust. Firstly, parents need to know these feelings are absolutely normal – to feel scared, anxious, worried. You're not being neurotic. Don't hide away from the allergy and don't take all the burden on yourself. Ask for support and spread the load. Look for help online too but you need to use sites where you can trust the information. Look for the information standard logo which is a guarantee the information has been clinically reviewed and is trustworthy.

How can parents stop their children becoming anxious about their allergies?

Talk to the children and involve them as early as possible. Some people want to shield them from anaphylaxis but it doesn't allow them to understand their condition or take ownership of it. Talk to your child, ask them how they feel. What is making them anxious? Look at how to help them manage it. Let them take their frustration out and help them to deal with their emotions. Say, we can't change it, but what can we do to make things better for you? Encourage them to be open about their condition.

What are the challenges for adults facing allergies?

Adults who develop allergies have to come to terms with managing something they never had to think about before. Now you have to ask questions, speak out, create a fuss. If you're restricting your life, it can create anxiety. There are lots of things you can do. If eating out makes you anxious, try to find places you can trust to be safe or where staff are very knowledgeable about allergies. Build up slowly. Have a trainer pen and remind yourself how to use it. There are different levels of support people need. A face to face, properly run support group is invaluable.

How can people manage their fears after a reaction?

It is important to try and look for positives after a reaction. What have you learnt? You know what happens and how to deal with it. The high anxiety you feel usually resolves over time but sometimes a reaction can be very scary and cause Post Traumatic Stress Disorder (PTSD) symptoms. Sometimes you need to say, 'I need more help.' Friends and family have good intentions but may not always know how to help. If you need more specialist help, try to find a therapist who knows about food allergies or is willing to understand it.

Chapter 16

NUTRITION, FOOD ELIMINATION AND REINTRODUCTION

When you or your child are first diagnosed with a food allergy, it can seem very daunting and overwhelming. You are suddenly faced with thinking about food in a completely different way. It is natural to feel nervous about questioning ingredients, understanding labels and finding alternatives.

The good news is, it is perfectly possible to have a full, varied and nutritionally complete diet while excluding multiple foods. Talk to a dietician about your individual nutritional requirements and how to address any gaps your particular allergy may present.

Milk

People with cow's milk allergy should avoid all dairy products including cheese, butter and yoghurt, unless they have passed a food challenge or have been told to trial reintroduction. Often milk is an added ingredient in many unsuspecting places including ham, bread and wine, so it is important to read labels carefully. Many people will also react to goat's and sheep's milk as the proteins are very similar so these should generally be avoided too.

Milk and dairy products are usually people's main source of calcium so it is important to include a fortified alternative, supplement or other dietary sources when you cut milk out. This is especially important for infants and breastfeeding mothers. (see: table 2 for calcium requirements or table 3 for calcium sources)

Egg

Eggs are unrelated to milk and dairy and are generally fairly easy to avoid in their whole form. Look for them as an ingredient in sausages, burgers or fresh pasta and you will probably need to avoid commercially baked goods too unless you have passed a food challenge or already tolerate them. It is safe to eat chicken if you have an egg allergy as the proteins in the flesh are different.

Wheat

Wheat is in many core foods we tend to rely on including bread, pasta and crackers. It can also often be found in sauces, spice mixes or condiments so be careful with labels. There are lots of alternative grains and many freefrom foods available. Remember, gluten is only a component of wheat and they are not the same thing. Gluten-free foods may still contain wheat, while other foods that contain gluten may be wheat free so be sure you check carefully.

Peanuts and tree nuts

Peanuts are not botanically classified as a nut but are actually a legume, along with peas, beans and lentils, while all other nuts – brazil, cashew almond etc. – are classified as tree nuts. Many people are allergic to peanuts but not tree nuts, while others may be allergic to some tree nuts but not others. Historically, many people have been told to avoid all nuts if they have an allergy to one, but recent studies suggest that keeping them in your diet may help prevent developing further allergies.

Coconut, nutmeg and pine nuts

There is often confusion about coconut, nutmeg and pine nuts because of their names, but they are not botanically nuts or legumes and do not need to be avoided unless you have a specific allergy to them.

Soya

Soya is a legume but most people with soya allergies can tolerate other beans and peanuts. Many infants with non-IgE cow's milk allergy will also react to soya as the proteins are very similar. A lot of products use soya lecithin as a stabiliser, but many people can tolerate this as the proteins are very low.

Sesame seeds

Some people are only allergic to sesame when the seeds are crushed – like in tahini, used in hummus – as this is when the majority of the proteins are released, whereas others will react to whole seeds used on bread or Asian dishes as well. There is no need to avoid any other seeds, unless you have a specific allergy to them.

Nut, seed and soy oils

Most nut, seed and soy oils used in cooking and cosmetics are safe as they have been highly refined and therefore the proteins which cause the allergic reactions have been removed. A small study involving 60 people with peanut allergy concluded that refined peanut oil posed no risk to any of those who took part. However, there have been reports of anaphylaxis to less refined oil, so it is important to be sure about an oil's composition before eating it and if in doubt, avoid it.

Lupin

Lupin is best known as a flower but the seeds of some varieties are also processed to make flour. They are a legume and the proteins are closely related to peanuts so may cause a similar reaction. The use of lupin flour in food is fairly rare so there is not much clinical evidence but some people with peanut allergies will also react to the similar proteins.

Celery

As well as avoiding the vegetable, people with celery allergy also need to avoid the seeds, spice and related root vegetable, celariac. Watch out for celery in stocks, sauces and flavourings. Reactions to celery can also be part of oral allergy syndrome.

Shellfish (crustaceans and molluscs)

There are two main groups of shellfish: crustaceans (crab, lobster, crayfish, prawns) and molluscs (e.g. mussels, oysters, scallops, octopus, squid). Most people who react to a shellfish in one of the groups will react to others in the same group. This doesn't mean they will necessarily react to shellfish in the other group though and it doesn't increase the likelihood of reacting to regular fish (e.g. cod, plaice etc) All shellfish has a high chance of cross-contamination though, especially on fish counters.

Fish

Fish are separate to shellfish and are usually categorised by having fins and scales. You may react to white fish (cod, seabass haddock) or oily fish (salmon, mackerel, trout) and be able to eat the other without any issues. Fish can often be hidden in sauces and salad dressings, and fish oil can often be a hidden ingredient in food and medication, so it is important to read ingredients carefully.

Mustard

As well as avoiding the condiment, it is important to check ingredients carefully as mustard is commonly used in many sauces, styles of cooking and also often added to processed foods. Some greens, mainly used in Asian cooking, are also from the mustard family.

Sulphites

Sulphites are a group of sulphur containing chemicals, including sulphur dioxide and sodium or potassium metabisulphite, better known as food preservatives (E220-228). They can be found in a lot of food and drink including wine, beer, soft drinks, sausages and frozen food. Most reactions to sulphites are a sensitivity rather than a true allergy and can exacerbate asthma or allergic rhinitis. It is rare to have an IgE mediated anaphylactic reaction.

Non-top 14 allergens

If you are allergic to a food that falls outside the top 14 and does not need to be labelled by law, it can be a little harder. There is less awareness and much less information available. You will need to read labels very carefully, talk about ingredients in detail if you eat out and help educate others. Watch out for anything labelled 'spices' or 'flavouring' as individual elements do not need to be listed.

Cross reactivity

There can be a lot of cross reactivity with food allergies, where you may react to foods that are in the same botanical group, but this is difficult to predict. For example, over 50 per cent of people allergic to one shellfish are likely to be allergic to another, while over 90 per cent of people with a peanut allergy can safely eat other legumes. Many people are allergic to one or more tree nuts but not others.

People with pollen allergies may suffer from Oral Allergy Syndrome as the proteins cross react with many raw fruits and vegetables (see: table 1), while it is relatively common for people with latex allergies to have problems with bananas and kiwi fruit, as these are also related.

Many people are dealing with multiple food allergies which can make their diets very restrictive. It is important to talk to a dietician or nutritionist about alternative sources of nutrients, substitutes and meal ideas. Once you get used to cooking and eating with food restrictions, it is amazing the number of dishes it is possible to make and how tasty vegan cakes or other alternatives can be.

It is important to maintain a healthy and balanced diet when you are dealing with food allergies and not limit your diet unnecessarily. Not only can this negatively impact your health, there is now evidence that excluding foods may lead to further allergies.

Food anxiety

Some people with food allergies may develop food anxiety as they associate eating with being ill. This can be very common in allergic children who are often more sensitive to tastes and textures or unwilling to try new foods for fear of a reaction. This can usually be combated by being patient, not pushing them and helping them get involved in preparing and cooking food, even if they won't eat it. More severe food aversions may need the help of a psychologist or play specialist to help you with strategies. In extreme cases, people may be put on an elemental formula diet to maintain nutrition while these issues are addressed.

'When I had lots of allergies I was scared of eating new things. I wanted to try things but I wasn't allowed. Now I can try new things. I'm really happy!'   *Ellie Knibb (5)*

Food elimination

If you have a suspected IgE-mediated reaction to a food then it is important to avoid it and contact your allergist or ask for a referral through your GP for testing. If the reactions are less well defined, for example you have non-IgE symptoms or suspect a food is exacerbating your eczema, then you will need to follow a careful elimination diet. This will help you understand what is causing your symptoms and stop you cutting out foods unnecessarily. You will need to cut a food out your diet for at least 2-4 weeks to see if there is any difference but many people will see results much quicker. It is best to only address one food at a time, so you can have a clear idea of whether it is causing your symptoms. Talk to your GP or a dietician about how to do this safely. If you are breastfeeding, it is important that any eliminations do not negatively affect your own health too.

Food challenges and reintroduction

If it is possible you or your child have outgrown an allergy or if you want to assess whether you are still reacting to it, then your doctor or dietician will encourage you to reintroduce it into your diet.

Any reintroductions should always be started under medical advice. If you or your child has had a serious reaction or shown high tests results in the past, then it is safer to do the first steps in hospital under a controlled food challenge (see more: chapter 6). After this, or if you are dealing with non-IgE allergies, you will probably be advised to carry out the reintroductions at home. You should only attempt reintroductions when you or your child is well, with no coughs or colds and any asthma is well under control. Children who introduce baked milk into their diet are up to more likely to become tolerant to all forms of cow's milk. Similarly children eating baked egg are more likely to become tolerant to regular egg, compared with children avoiding all forms. The same studies showed children regularly eating baked egg products also tolerated regular egg on average 2-2.5 years earlier.[1]

> 'I felt happy when I could have dairy again because it's so yummy and I don't have to be scared any more.'   *Theo Wood (5)*

Milk ladder

Cow's milk is the most common childhood allergy and 80 per cent of children will outgrow it by preschool age. There is a reintroduction programme called the milk ladder which can be used under the guidance of a doctor or dietician to help reintroduce milk, using foods that slowly increase the levels of proteins. Depending on previous reactions, you may be given varying timescales of how quickly to tackle each stage.

For children with non-IgE allergies, it is usually advised to start trying the milk ladder after a child's first birthday. For children with IgE-mediated allergies, it will depend more on whether test results have reduced or if they have passed a hospital food challenge. However, up to 75% people can tolerate baked milk (in biscuits or cakes) before they can tolerate butter, yoghurt or fresh milk. This is because the proteins are broken down so much in the heating process. Therefore, your allergist may suggest you attempt a baked milk challenge, even if test results are still positive.

For mothers who are still breastfeeding, it is possible to introduce the foods into your own diet first to see if your baby reacts by following the same steps. You may also find you have built up an intolerance to cow's milk by excluding it from your diet, so it can help to reintroduce it slowly too.

Egg ladder

The next most common allergy to grow out of is egg. Again, up to 80 per cent of children will outgrow this before they start school.

Like milk, many people can tolerate baked egg because the proteins are extensively broken down in the cooking process. This means you may be able to eat it in cakes with no reactions, while still being allergic to it in an omelette.

There is a similar 'ladder' that is used to help slowly introduce egg into your or your child's diet under the guidance of your doctor or dietician. If there is a history of a severe reaction, then your doctor may suggest completing a egg challenge in a hospital setting.

Introducing other foods

A similar process can be followed for many other foods, although the steps are often less well defined. Your doctor or dietician will be able to advise you further.

Desensitisation

Once you or your child can tolerate a food at any level, then it is important to keep it in your diet on a regular basis – at least twice a week. This will help the body continue to tolerate it. Some allergy clinics encourage desensitisation by very slowly increasing these amounts. For example, if you fail a food challenge you may continue eating the amount you tolerated (for example, half a baked egg muffin) regularly at home and slowly and carefully increase this over time to a full muffin. Talk to your allergist about whether this approach may be beneficial and safe for you.

> Although I knew you could outgrow an allergy and had read about it, Ellie's reactions were so severe, even to touch, that I didn't dare thinking she'd outgrow them. Ellie's first reaction occurred when I started weaning her at 5 months. She is now 5 years old and food challenges have now confirmed she has outgrown her allergies to soya, milk protein, wheat and baked egg.' *Mel Knibb*

Expert Insight: Food allergies and nutrition

Rosan Meyer
Paediatric dietician

What are the main nutritional deficiencies you see with food allergies?

If the diet is well managed, there are very few nutritional needs that cannot be met, even when avoiding the top allergens. The problem is when people aren't informed and don't get the proper advice. If there is a delay in weaning and babies are missing iron rich proteins, then we often see a lack of iron. Or, for example if you are vegetarian and have a legume allergy, it can become difficult to manage due to risk of deficiencies. Vitamin D is very important and you can only get about 10 per cent of the recommended daily amount through diet so a supplement (as per Department of Health Requirements) or fortified milk is very important.

Many mums go on exclusion diets when breastfeeding allergic babies. How can these be best managed?

It can be very difficult when you are breastfeeding a baby with allergies. Allergens like milk, egg, wheat and soya do transfer through breast milk, but as such a dietary elimination is very challenging it is best done with the guidance of a dietitian. In the majority of cases it's only one or two allergens that are the culprits and we do not want to risk unnecessarily taking all of the allergens out and impacting on the mum's nutritional status and her quality of life. Breastfeeding has many benefits and mothers should try to breast feed if possible and access support. The only time to consider stopping is if there is harm done to either mother or baby; if your child is continuing to lose weight or if you have lost weight beyond your pre-pregnancy weight, if it harmful for the psychological wellbeing of the mother or leading to a vitamin of mineral deficiency in mother or child.

How can parents approach weaning to minimise the risk of allergic reaction or to identify allergenic foods?

Introduce the least allergenic foods first (i.e. vegetables, fruit) and try new foods every three days. Introduce them well cooked before giving raw, as cooking reduces allergenicity and try them at the beginning of the day. Try to give them a few teaspoons before trying baby led feeding as it is easier to know what they have eaten and how much. Food diaries can be problematic in trying to identify allergens, as you can get both delayed reactions (it can take days for reactions to occur) and symptoms can become worse due to other factors outside of food introductions, including teething or having a cold.

Does reintroducing baked milk and egg help a child outgrow their allergy?

If a child can tolerate baked egg or milk (as judged by a healthcare professional) then it is more likely they will outgrow that allergy. Studies are still looking at whether this is due to them building a tolerance through their body accepting the baked version or if those who tolerate baked are less allergic to begin with.

Are they any ways, beyond early introduction, that parents can help prevent their children developing allergies?

Giving your child home cooked food helps improve gut microbiota diversity, which some studies have indicated plays a role in the development of allergies. There is also some evidence coming though that some specific probiotics could help prevent atopic dermatitis and improve tolerance to cow's milk. It may be worth discussing this with your healthcare professional as an option.

Chapter 17

PREVENTING ALLERGIES

The understanding of allergies, how they develop and why the body attacks different proteins is growing all the time. There has been some high-profile research in the last few years looking at how allergies develop and ways to reduce them in infants. There are more studies taking place exploring this further and also delving deeper into the link between allergies and the microbiome. There is still currently no cure or categoric way to prevent allergies but there are a lot of avenues that may prove invaluable.

The eczema link

A leading theory is that many infants develop food allergies after being sensitised by proteins entering their body through the skin before they have eaten them. This is more likely to happen if the skin is broken, for example when a child has eczema.

Research found that infants were more likely to develop a peanut allergy in households with high environmental exposure to peanut, through family members eating them, unless the infant had consumed peanut in the first year of life.[1]

Therefore, preventing eczema through emollient use from birth and quickly and effectively treating any flare ups, may help prevent this early sensitisation. There are also small-scale studies that suggest this may be true for environmental allergens too.

Breastfeeding

The other area of research that is becoming prevalent is the link between gut health and developing allergies. It is suggested that the stronger and more diverse someone's microbiome – the microorganisms in the body - the less likely they are to develop allergies.

The use of antibiotics in early life has long been seen as a risk factor for developing allergies as it disrupts the microbiome. So has being born by caesarean section, as babies do not get the same protective bacteria from their mother as during a vaginal birth.

One way to help counter this is through exclusive breastfeeding until 6 months which helps build a baby's immune system. Breastmilk transfers beneficial bacteria from the mother to increase and strengthen the diversity of the child's microbiome.[2] Some studies suggest this difference in protective bacteria lasts until the child is seven and can also help prevent children developing asthma.[3]

Probiotics

Research shows that allergic children have different intestinal gut flora to non-allergic children with less probiotic bacteria present.[4] This healthy probiotic bacteria can help children develop immune tolerance, while those without it have a higher chance of developing allergies.[5] In a study which looked at women taking probiotics during pregnancy and in the first three months of breastfeeding, the incidence of food allergies in children at 2 years old was reduced significantly.[6]

There is no clear evidence whether introducing probiotics at a later stage can help children outgrow allergies or build tolerance. However, Lactobacillus GG probiotics were recently used alongside immunotherapy in the PPOIT (Probiotic with peanut oral immunotherapy) trial in Australia with promising results.

Fish oil

Taking fish oil containing Omega-3 fatty acids during pregnancy and the first few months of breastfeeding may also help prevent allergies, although you should always discuss this with your doctor or midwife first. Research at Imperial College London, which looked at nineteen different trials, found this could reduce eggs allergies at age one by 30 per cent. The same study found that taking probiotics could also reduce eczema in infants by 20 per cent.

Vitamin D

A number of studies have shown a link between food allergies and a lack of vitamin D. A study in Australia mapped where children with allergies lived and found a strong correlation with them being in the less sunny south of the country.[7] Research also suggests more children with allergies are born in autumn and winter.[8] There is no direct evidence to show increasing vitamin D in pregnancy or early life can help prevent allergies, but studies suggest it may have a beneficial effect.

Early food introduction

It used to be believed that the best way to prevent allergies was to avoid highly allergenic food during pregnancy and early life. However, researchers looked into regional variations and found that peanut allergies are more common in the UK than in a genetically similar population in Israel, where peanut-containing foods are eaten at an earlier age.[9]

Two significant studies – EAT (Enquiring About Tolerance) and LEAP (Learning Early About Peanut Allergy) – have looked further into this and turned the previous advice on its head. It is now believed that introducing these foods between 4-11 months can actually prevent children from developing allergies to them.

The LEAP study looked at infants who were at high risk of developing peanut allergy due to a history of moderate or severe eczema and/or an egg allergy in early life. They were then put in a group who either introduced and regularly ate peanuts from between 4-11 months of age until 5 years old or avoided them completely for the same period. The study found that 81 per cent fewer children developed peanut allergies in the group who consumed them regularly. It also found that sensitisation to food allergens can occur as early as 3-4 months, so the introduction is more effective earlier in infancy.

The EAT study looked at whether introducing the most allergenic foods regularly to infants from 3 months, alongside continued breastfeeding, could reduce the prevalence of food allergies by 3 years old. The study showed no cases of anaphylaxis during the initial introduction and no adverse effects on breastfeeding or growth.

The study found that it was difficult for participants to stick strictly to the protocol and continue to feed regular amounts of each food to their child. However, out of those who did stick strictly to the criteria (42 per cent) it showed significant results. By the age of three, 2.5 percent of children in the avoidance group had peanut allergies compared to no children in the group who ate them regularly. It also found 5.5 per cent of children who avoided eggs developed an allergy, compared to just 1.4 per cent who introduced them early.

'When our baby showed signs of cow's milk allergy and eczema, I sought a referral to a paediatrician as early as possible to try and get advice before we started introducing solids. Our paediatrician conducted a skin prick test for major allergens, and when it was negative, recommended that we introduce peanuts and egg as early as possible and feed them to him regularly due to a strong family history of allergy. As this is such new guidance we had to feel our own way a little bit with how to do this. We found the best way has been to mix smooth peanut butter into his breakfast cereal, or have peanut puffs or peanut butter on toast as a finger food. I still feel a bit anxious about giving egg as that's his big sister's allergy and I feed him boiled egg once a week when she's at nursery.' *Carly Talbot.*

Expert Insight: Preventing allergies in infants

Professor George Du Toit, Paediatric Allergy Consultant
Mary Feeney, Clinical research dietician

How can parents practically apply the LEAP findings at home?

Once their baby is established on some of the typical first infant foods, they can also introduce peanut. They can use smooth peanut butter, mixing a teaspoonful with 2-3 teaspoons of warm water or baby's milk until it's a thinner, smooth texture. This can be given as it is or mixed with other foods like pureed or mashed fruit, vegetables, baby's porridge, or yoghurt. They can also use puffed peanut products such as Bamba which are a soft texture that dissolves in the mouth. Babies can eat these from around 7 months. If they are eating peanut foods and tolerating them well, they should be continued around twice a week, giving about a rounded teaspoon of peanut butter, 20g grams of puffed peanut snacks or about 10 peanuts ground to a powder.

Are there any risks of early introduction and how can these be managed?

There is a risk that some children will react on the first occasion they eat peanut. Parents should discuss with their GP, paediatrician or allergist about precautionary screening or medications e.g. antihistamines which they could use to treat an immediate reaction. However, it is also important that waiting for screening allergy tests does not unnecessarily delay the introduction of allergen foods which can increase the risk of developing allergy.

If an infant has a milk allergy or reactions to other foods, should parents still introduce peanuts early?

If the infant has a cow's milk allergy and no other allergy symptoms or diagnosis, they should introduce solids at around 6 months of age including the common allergens. Peanut should be introduced during the first year of life.

If the infant has a known risk factor for food allergy e.g. eczema in the first three months of life, and/or an egg allergy and their baby is showing signs of readiness for solids, they should consider introducing solids including cooked egg and then peanut between 4-6 months followed by the other food allergens; ideally alongside continued breastfeeding. If their child has an immediate type, IgE-mediated food allergy referral to a specialist allergy clinic is recommended.

How should this be approached when a parent has a peanut allergy?

A family history of food allergy, including peanut allergy, is no longer considered an important risk factor for an individual developing peanut allergy. If introducing peanut to an infant in a household where there is someone who already has a peanut allergy, precautions will need to be taken to protect this person from reacting e.g. feeding peanut only in one location such as a high chair, and ensuring thorough cleaning of utensils, surfaces and the infant's hands and face after the feeding. This could be discussed with a healthcare professional.

Does this early introduction apply to tree nuts and other allergens too?

The Pronuts Study has finished a feasibility study and anticipates commencing a prospective randomized controlled trial. Their research is looking at the question of whether regular introduction of specific 'safe' nuts and seeds (those the child has been tested and confirmed tolerant to at the start of the study) will prevent spread and worsening of peanut, tree-nut and sesame seed allergies.

There is also some evidence from the EAT study that the introduction of cooked egg in the first year of life is effective to prevent the development of egg allergy.

How effective is the same exposure for older children?

We are not sure as yet. The Pronuts Study is looking at the development of allergies in children aged 0-16 years. We noted on the LEAP Study that older infants had higher allergy test results which suggests that children who have the risk factors for developing peanut allergy have a greater likelihood of already being allergic the older they are, this is why we encourage the introduction of peanut early.

Chapter 18

LIVING WITH ALLERGIES

L iving with allergies can be frustrating, upsetting and can make things people take for granted difficult, painful or even life threatening. However, the more you get used to them and learn to manage them effectively, the more it is possible to lead a full and fun life. You may have to do things a little differently but here are my top tips for not letting your allergies hold you back:

Do your research. The more you understand about your individual allergies the easier it is to address them. Get a referral to an allergist and talk to them in detail, taking along a list of any questions. Read books, articles and research papers online so you are armed with all the facts.

Trust your instinct. You know yourself or your child best. It can be hard when you are getting conflicting information or a lack of support from medical professionals but keep going until you get the answers you need.

Always be prepared. Planning ahead is the key to going out and about with allergies. Check menus, venues or activities well in advance and talk to hosts, teachers or friends about how you may need to address things. Carry your medication, pack safe snacks and be sure any caregivers know what to do in an emergency.

Take small steps. Do not force yourself into situations you find difficult but try to take small steps to widen your comfort zone. This will make you feel more confident and in control. Talk to others who live with allergies and learn from their experiences.

Think positively. Try to focus on the things you can do, rather than the things you can't.

Look for solutions. There will be plenty of challenges along the way but instead of letting them get you down, try and find ways around them. There is usually a different way to do something. It may take extra work or planning and you might not get it right first time, but keep trying.

Build your support network. Living with allergies can be lonely and isolating so it is important you have support. This may be from friends and family who you have educated about your allergies, or from people who deal with allergies themselves. Online forums can be a great way to connect with others, but nothing beats meeting up in person.

Be kind to yourself. Allergies can take a lot out of you, mentally and physically. So if you are feeling anxious or overwhelmed, try to be gentle on yourself and do something to relax or have fun. Stay as healthy as possible to support your body and seek help if you need to.

I hope this book has given you some more information and insight into living with allergies, along with lots of tips you can put into practice. Everyone's journey is different and your experiences, needs and challenges may change as your allergies do or during different times of your life.

My two allergic children are the reason I have delved into the subject of allergies, started my blog and written this book. They inspire me every day with their love, enthusiasm and ability to live in the present. Their allergies are part of who they are and have already helped positively shape their empathy, confidence and maturity.

We are still relatively early on our allergy journey and I am still hopeful they may grow out some of them or have access to immunotherapies in the future. If they don't though, I want them to know that they can lead a full life without letting their allergies hold them back.

Come and join us!

Visit our blog www.freefromfarmhouse.co.uk to find recipes, advice and more insight into how our family live with allergies. Or to connect with other people living with allergies, in a positive and supportive environment, join our Facebook group
www.facebook.com/groups/livingwithallergies

TABLES

Table 1: Oral Allergy Syndrome

	Common	**Less common**
Fruit	Apple Peach Pear Plum Cherry Nectarine Apricot Kiwi Strawberry	Orange Melon Watermelon Mango Pineapple
Vegetables	Carrot Celery Peeling potatoes Soy milk Tomato	Swiss chard Beans and peas Mange tout Bean sprouts Parsley Fennel Cucumber Peppers Courgettes
Nuts/Peanuts	Hazelnut Almond Walnut Brazil nut	Peanuts
Spices		Coriander Cumin Aniseed Caraway Mustard Sunflower seeds

Table 2: Calcium requirements

Age	Daily RNI (Reference Nutrient Intake)
0-12 months (non-breastfed only)	525mg
1-3 years	350mg
4-6 years	450mg
7-10 years	550mg
11-18 years – boys	1000mg
11-18 years – girls	800mg
Adults (19+) years	700mg
Pregnant women	700mg
Breastfeeding women	700mg + 550mg

Table 3: Non-dairy calcium sources

200ml calcium fortified non-dairy milk	200mg
125g calcium-fortified soya yoghurt	200mg
120g tofu	200mg
50g sardines	200mg
200g baked beans	100mg
1tsp tahini	100mg
110g broccoli	50mg
8 dried apricots	50mg
1 large orange	50mg
I medium slice bread	50mg
10 almonds	50mg

Table 4: RAST test IgE level results

Rast rating/class	IgE level (KUI/L)	
0	< 0.35	Absent/undetectable
1	0.35 – 0.7	Low
2	0.7 – 3.5	Medium
3	3.5 – 17.5	High
4	17.5 – 50	Very High
5	50 – 100	Very High
6	>100	Extremely High

RESOURCES

Guidelines

Allergy UK: Resources for schools
www.allergyuk.org/information-and-advice/for-schools/useful-allergy-resources-for-schools

Allergy UK: Food diary
www.allergyuk.org/get-help/resources/321-food-symptoms-diary

BSACI: Paediatric allergy action plans
www.bsaci.org/about/download-paediatric-allergy-action-plans

BSACI: find an allergist
www.bsaci.org

British Psychological Society: find a psychologist
www.bps.org.uk/public/find-psychologist

Discrimination Disability Act
www.gov.uk/definition-of-disability-under-equality-act-2010

iMap patient factsheet
www.allergyuk.org/assets/000/001/299/iMAP_Patient_Factsheet_original.pdf

MHRA adrenaline auto-injector review
www.gov.uk/drug-safety-update/adrenaline-auto-injectors-updated-advice-after-european-review

NICE: Cow's milk allergy in children
https://cks.nice.org.uk/cows-milk-protein-allergy-in-children

NICE: Drug allergy diagnosis and management
www.nice.org.uk/guidance/cg183

NICE: Food allergy pathway in under 19s
https://www.nice.org.uk/guidance/cg116

Guidance on the use of adrenaline auto-injectors in school – Department of health and social care
www.gov.uk/government/publications/using-emergency-adrenaline-auto-injectors-in-schools

Supporting pupils at school with medical conditions - Department for Education
www.gov.uk/government/publications/supporting-pupils-at-school-with-medical-conditions--3

Useful websites

Allergy UK
www.allergyuk.org
01322 619898
The UK's leading allergy charity offers advice, support and a helpline.

Allergy Adventures
www.allergyadventures.com/
Fun and educational resources for children, and school workshops.

Allergy Buddies
www.allergybuddies.com
Personalised child friendly allergy alert products.

Allergic Living
www.allergicliving.com
American magazine for people living with allergies and asthma.

Allergy Lifestyle
www.allergylifestyle.com
Online store for allergy and asthma products. Ships worldwide.

Allergy and asthma network (US website)
www.allergyasthmanetwork.org/
American non-profit organisation working to end needless suffering and death from allergies and asthma.

Allergy Wise
www.allergywise.org.uk
Online allergy training courses from Anaphylaxis Campaign

Anaphylaxis campaign
www.anaphylaxis.org.uk
UK charity supporting people with severe allergies and anaphylaxis. Run in person support groups.

Allergy Travels
www.allergytravels.com
Helping people with allergies travel safely and confidently.

Asthma UK
www.asthma.org.uk
Providing advice and support for people living with asthma.

Cambridge Peanut Allergy Clinic
www.peanut.cuh.org.uk/
Private allergy clinic offering peanut immunotherapy.

Disability Living Allowance
www.gov.uk/disability-living-allowance-children
Some children with complex health conditions may be eligible for disability living allowance.

Free From Food Awards
www.freefromfoodawards.co.uk/
Find the best allergy friendly food products on the market

Free From Eating Out Awards
www.freefromeatingoutawards.co.uk/
Find the best allergy friendly places to eat out in the UK.

FPIES Foundation
www.fpiesfoundation.org/
American organisation supporting peopole with FPIES

Food Allergy Research And Education
www.foodallergy.org/
World's largest non-profit organisation providing research, education and support for people with food allergies.

Food Standards Agency
www.food.gov.uk/
Information about food allergens, labelling, eating out and how to report a problem.

Haydn's Wish
www.haydns-wish.co.uk/
Raising awareness of the link between asthma and allergies in children.

Kyle Dine Music
www.kyledine.com/
Food allergy awareness songs for children

Met Office: pollen forecast
www.metoffice.gov.uk/public/weather/pollen-forecast/

Apps

Allergy translation
www.allergytranslation.com
Order allergy translation cards in over 40 languages that you can print off or store on your phone.

Alert 5
www.alert5.co.uk/
Alert 5 people of your exact location if you need urgent assistance.

Food Maestro
www.foodmaestro.me/food-app/
Developed in partnership with Guys a nd St Thomas Hospital, this app allows you set up a profile with your food allergies, scan labels and find safe products.

Spoon Guru
www.spoon.guru/the-app/
Find new foods and recipes based on your dietary requirements.

Books

HEGGIE, Fiona & **LUX**, Ellie, *Allergy free baby and toddler cookbook*, Orion 2016
Recipes for weaning and toddlers, free from top 14 allergens.

HEGGIE, Fiona & **LUX**, Ellie, *Allergy free family cookbook*, Orion 2015.
Family recipes free from most of the top allergens with lots of easy substitutions

POMPA, Robin Nixon, *Allergy free kids: The science based approach to preventing food allergies,* William Morrow 2017
Advice and recipes for introducing allergens to children

SICHERER, Scott H, *Food allergies: a complete guide to eating when your life depends on it (2nd edition)*John Hopkins University Press 2017
Detailed and practical book answering numerous questions about the science of food allergies.

WAGGOTT, Jamie, *Tom's Secret Agents,* Create Space 2014
An illustrated book written by a young boy about living with a nut allergy. It's fun and easy to understand. For 3-8yr olds

Blogs

Allergy Girl Eats
www.allergygirleats.com
Recipes and advice for living as an adult with multiple allergies.

Dairy Free Kids
www.dairyfreekids.ie
Shopping, cooking and living with dairy free kids.

Dilan And Me
www.dilanandme.com
Living and breastfeeding with milk and soy allergies.

Eat Allergy Safe
www.eatallergysafe.com
Blog and podcast offering advice about living with allergies.

Intolerant Gourmand
www.intolerantgourmand.com
Recipes and advice for raising a child with multiple allergies.

Miss Allergic Reactor
www.missallergicreactor.com
Lifestyle and travel tips for living with allergies and asthma.

The Peachicks' Bakery
www.thepeachicksbakery.co.uk
Dairy free, gluten free and vegan recipes.

What Allergy
www.whatallergy.com
Advice and insight into living as an adult with allergies, asthma and eczema.

Online support groups

Allergy Travels
www.facebook.com/groups/allergytravels

Breastfeeding with Cow's milk protein (CMPA) and other food allergies
www.facebook.com/groups/breastfeedingwithCMPA

Cow's milk protein allergy (CMPA) support
www.facebook.com/groups/Allergy.diet

Living with allergies
www.facebook.com/groups/livingwithallergies

Official Allergy UK support group
www.facebook.com/groups/officialallergyuksupportgroup/

ENDNOTES

Chapter 1: Understanding Allergies

1. Hourihane J (2006) The prevalence of peanut allergy in British children at school entry age in 2003.
2. Ownby DR. Environmental factors versus genetic determinants of childhood inhalants allergies. *Journal of Allergy and Clinical Immunology.* 1990; 86:279–87
3. Shared genetic origin of asthma, hay fever and eczema elucidates allergic disease biology
4. Gupta R et al. (2007) *Thorax* 162:91-96
5. Mintel, 2010
6. Nwaru BI & Group., 2014
7. Vassallo MF, Banerji A, Rudders SA et al. Season of birth and food-induced anaphylaxis in Boston. Allergy. 2010;65(11):1492–3.
8. Branum A, Lukacs S. Food allergy among U.S. children: Trends in prevalence and hospitalizations. NCHS data brief, no 10. Hyattsville, MD: National Center for Health Statistics. 2008.
9. Wlasiuk G & Vercelli D (2012) Current Opinion in Allergy and Clinical Immunology 12:461-466

Chapter 2: Food Allergies

1. National Institute for Health and Clinical Excellence, 2011
2. Venter, C., Pereira, B., Voigt, K., Grundy, J., Clayton, C. B., Higgins, B., Arshad, S. H. and Dean, T. (2009). Factors associated with maternal dietary intake, feeding and weaning practices, and the development of food hypersensitivity in the infant. *Pediatric Allergy and Immunology.* 20: 320-327.

Chapter 3: Environmental And Other Allergies

1. House dust mite exposure as a cause of asthma. [*Clinical and Experimental Allergy*. 1993]
2. https://www.nice.org.uk/guidance/cg183/chapter/introduction

Chapter 5: Respiratory Allergies

1. Asthma UK, 2017
2. Simonte SJ, et al. Relevance of casual contact with peanut butter in children with peanut allergy. Journal of Allergy and Clinical Immunology.. 2003 Jul:112 (1): 180-2.
3. Pawankar R, et al, 2013

Chapter 8: Allergy Medication

1. Allergy and Asthma network
2. Determining the Efficacy and Value of Immunotherapy on the Likelihood of Peanut Tolerance: The DEVIL Study (DEVIL)

Chapter 9: Allergies In Infants

1. BSACI, 2011
2. Pawankar R, et al, 2013

Chapter 15: Support and psychological effects

1. EAACI 2016

Chapter 16: Nutrition, Food Elimination And Reintroduction

http://www.londonallergy.com/what-we-treat/food-allergies/

Chapter 17: Preventing Allergies

1. Du Toit G et al. (2008) *Journal of Allergy and Clinical Immunology*
2. Probiotics in Pregnant Women to Prevent Allergic Disease: A Randomized, Double-blind Trial – C.K. Dotterud; O. Storrø; R. Johnsen; T. Øien
3. Kalliomäki M, Kirjavainen P, Eerola E, et al. Distinct patterns of neonatal gut microflora in infants developing or not developing atopy. *Journal of Allergy and ClinicalImmunology*2001;107:129–34.
4. Various effects of different probiotic strains in allergic disorders: an update from laboratory and clinical data – Ö Özdemir

5. Probiotics in Asthma and Allergy Prevention – Maurizio Mennini, Lamia Dahdah, Maria Cristina Artesani, Alessandro Fiocchi, and Alberto Martelli

6. Association Between Breast Milk Bacterial Communities and Establishment and Development of the Infant Gut Microbiome Pia S. Pannaraj, MD, MPH1,2; Fan Li, PhD1; Chiara Cerini, MD1; et al

7. Mullins R.J., Clark S, Camargo C.A. Jr (2009). Regional variation in epinephrine autoinjector prescriptions in Australia: more evidence for the vitamin D-anaphylaxis hypothesis. *Annals of Allergy and Asthma Immunology*.103(6):488-95.)

8. Vassallo M.F., Banerji A., Rudders S.A. et al. Season of birth and food-induced anaphylaxis in Boston. Allergy. 2010;65(11):1492–3.

9. Du Toit G et al. (2008) *Journal of Allergy and Clinical Immunology*

INDEX